Twelve Hours' Sleep

by

Twelve Weeks Old

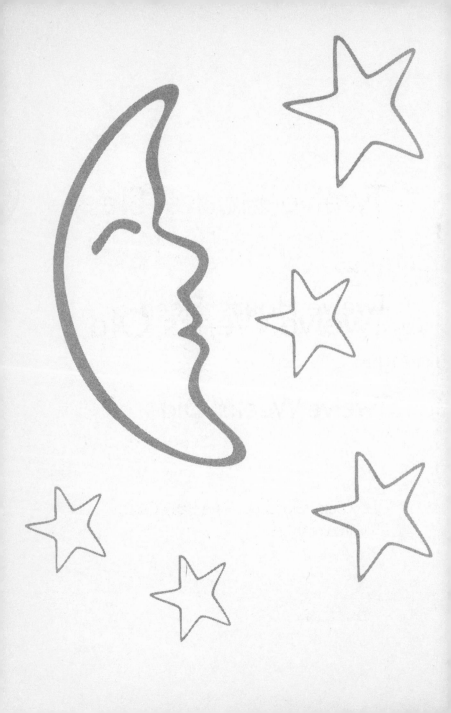

Twelve Hours' Sleep

by

Twelve Weeks Old

A Step-by-Step Plan for Baby Sleep Success

by Suzy Giordano, "The Baby Coach"
with Lisa Abidin

DUTTON

DUTTON
Published by Penguin Group (USA) Inc.
375 Hudson Street, New York, New York 10014, U.S.A.
Penguin Group (Canada), 90 Eglinton Avenue East, Suite 700, Toronto, Ontario M4P
2Y3, Canada (a division of Pearson Penguin Canada Inc.); Penguin Books Ltd,
80 Strand, London WC2R 0RL, England; Penguin Ireland, 25 St Stephen's Green,
Dublin 2, Ireland (a division of Penguin Books Ltd); Penguin Group (Australia), 250
Camberwell Road, Camberwell, Victoria 3124, Australia (a division of Pearson
Australia Group Pty Ltd); Penguin Books India Pvt Ltd, 11 Community Centre,
Panchsheel Park, New Delhi – 110 017, India; Penguin Group (NZ), cnr Airborne and
Rosedale Roads, Albany, Auckland 1310, New Zealand (a division of Pearson New
Zealand Ltd); Penguin Books (South Africa) (Pty) Ltd, 24 Sturdee Avenue, Rosebank,
Johannesburg 2196, South Africa

Penguin Books Ltd, Registered Offices: 80 Strand, London WC2R 0RL, England

Published by Dutton, a member of Penguin Group (USA) Inc.

First printing, January 2006
30 29 28 27 26 25 24 23

The information contained here is not intended to replace the advice that you should
receive from your doctor or other qualified health professional. Every infant is different, and variations in care may be recommended based on individual circumstances.

Z REGISTERED TRADEMARK—MARCA REGISTRADA

LIBRARY OF CONGRESS CATALOGING-IN-PUBLICATION DATA HAS BEEN APPLIED FOR.

ISBN 0-525-94959-3

Printed in the United States of America
Designed by Jaime Putorti

While the author has made every effort to provide accurate telephone numbers and
Internet addresses at the time of publication, neither the publisher nor the author as-
sumes any responsibility for errors, or for changes that occur after publication. Further, publisher does not have any control over and does not assume any responsibility
for author or third-party Web sites or their content.

To my children, Camilla, Bruno, Marcella, Thiago, and Matheus, who have taught me all the lessons that have led to this book. It is an honor to be called your mother. For the love, understanding, and a great journey I thank you!

—*Suzy Giordano*

For my children, Lauren and Michael Jr., and my husband, Michael Sr. Without all of you, this book would not exist. I love you always.

—*Lisa Abidin*

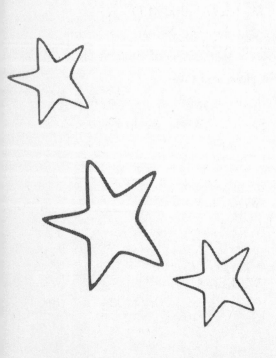

Contents

Contents

Foreword

"You better get some sleep!" Haunting words tossed out at soon-to-be parents. Lisa and I heard it many times, especially since we were expecting twins. We were lucky enough to have help at night and we were lucky enough to meet Suzy.

I heard Suzy and Lisa talk endlessly about raising babies. Very early on, I heard the claim of twelve hours' sleep by twelve weeks for twins, even less for singletons. Suzy casually mentioned the possibility of writing a book and I immediately jumped on the idea. She returned the next night to find a tape recorder, dictation machine, and laptop computer. Between Suzy and Lisa, the perfect marriage for a book was made. Suzy brought her wisdom of the ancients, raw empiricism, and bountiful common sense and blended it with Lisa's own recent experience training our babies using Suzy's methods and her ability to craft the concepts into a step-by-step "cookbook" type text.

As a medical doctor, I searched the common sources to ensure that our babies would receive enough nutrition from their feedings to sustain and maintain growth. The Merck manual reports that an infant should receive 50–55 kcal per pound per day. The method employed herein requires that the child weigh at least nine pounds and consume at least 24 ounces of formula or breast milk a day. Twenty-four ounces of standard formula provides a volume of 720 ml at a concentration of 0.67 kcal per ounce, or a total of 482.4 kcal. This divided by nine pounds equals 53.3 kcal per pound, and is right in line with the Merck recommendation. I was struck by the homology involved as it became apparent that Suzy had worked out the perfect amount of nutrition needed to sleep through the night by trial and error. It also made me wonder if those who worked out the weights and measures in earlier times also stumbled upon this measurement; 1 ounce per hour. As the child grows, the amount of food is increased and other foods are later introduced in order to meet the increasing nutritional demands of the child. Children do thrive under this plan, as borne out by Suzy's years of experience. Medicine has shown that children release growth hormones during sleep, and, therefore, sleep plays an important part in childhood growth.

In short, the plan works. Children are content. Parents are happy. The household is a calmer and more nurturing environment.

I am delighted to have had a small part in something I feel will add so much to the lives of parents and their children.

—*Michael Abidin, M.D.*

Twelve Hours' Sleep

by

Twelve Weeks Old

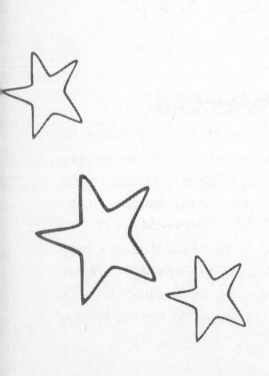

Introduction

✳ My Background ✳

By the time I was 26 years old I had five children, the youngest being fraternal twin boys. When my twins were born, I had an eight-year-old daughter, a seven-year-old son, and a two-year-old daughter. At that point in my life, I had no idea I would one day be a Baby Coach. I was as overwhelmed as you might imagine anyone would be. I am originally from Brazil, and the culture there is very different from that in the U.S. when it comes to bearing the responsibilities of raising children. Moms and aunts do not come for the first three weeks to help out while women recover from delivery. Most husbands have never changed a single diaper in their lives, much less stayed awake to help with nighttime feedings. Cloth diapers were the norm, and there was no outside company to pick up and deliver them fresh and clean to your home. To add insult to injury, there was also no washing machine or dryer. Wives cooked homemade meals from scratch at least three times a day. And by scratch, I mean no L'eggo my Eggo, no Wonder bread, no Newman's Own.

The first weeks of my life after my twins were born went something like this: I tried to breastfeed them every two hours, but I had very little milk coming in (about ½ ounce per feeding). In addition, I was changing 14–20 diapers a day (well, really 56–80 diapers if you count the fact that each child wore four cloth diapers at a time. Cloth diapers are much thinner in Brazil than they are here), hand-washing them in my kitchen sink, and hanging them on a line to dry outside or oftentimes draped around the bathroom, since it rains a lot in Brazil. I was also cleaning the twins' clothes, as well as my two year old's, my seven year old's, my eight year old's, my husband's, and mine. All by hand, all without a dryer. I was also preparing three full meals a day, completely from scratch, for five people as well as doing the normal day-to-day housekeeping.

Catering to the needs of seven people with about 45 minutes of sleep each night lasted about three weeks. I arrived desperate at my parents' home one morning at 5:00 AM. My dad said he would watch the twins for a couple of hours so I could get some sleep. I went to bed only to wake again to the crowing rooster, but found the sun was still not up. I thought I must have drifted off for about 15 minutes, but could not go back to sleep, so I went out to check on the twins. There was my dad feeding them bottled formula. I said, "Oh, I couldn't sleep, so you can hand them over to me." My dad looked puzzled, and then said, "Suzy, what do you mean? I have been feeding them all day and all night. You have been asleep for 24 hours."

At that point my dad sat me down and told me, "You cannot go on living like this, you have to develop a plan." And on that day I did develop a plan, a plan that my twins were still following when I emigrated from Brazil to Virginia in 1990. My twins were a year old, and a friend of a friend, Sarah, who had six-month-old triplets, came to visit one night. She gazed in jaw-dropping glory as she watched my twins with blankies in hand kiss us good night and start crawling up the stairs to their beds. She asked how long they had been doing this, and I told her since they were about three months old. At this point she asked if I could help her do the same with her triplets.

Sarah's life at home had become chaotic. She went from a home that consisted of her, her husband, and three pets to adding four day nannies, three night nannies, an au pair, a housekeeper and, most importantly, three babies (two girls and one boy) who were up all night. There were three different shifts of workers, working seven days a week, twenty-four hours a day. Needless to say, Sarah and her husband were finding it difficult to transition from their quiet DINK (Double Income No Kids) lifestyle to the literal three-ring circus their life had become.

When I went to Sarah's home for the first time, I told her it would be easy to train her babies to sleep through the night. She then asked me to help her, saying, "Where am I going to find someone who is going to do what you are telling me can be done?"

Point well taken. Even today, despite the numerous baby books and baby services available, you will not find a lot of entries in the Yellow Pages under "Baby Sleep Specialist." And for the handful of us who do train infants to sleep through the night, the demand far exceeds the supply.

After three weeks I had trained the triplets to sleep twelve hours at night with a one-hour nap in the morning and a two-hour nap in the afternoon. Sarah went from a staff of nine down to just one au pair. Sarah belonged to a Washington, D.C., area triplet club and told her "little sister" in the club, Leah, about me. I took care of Leah's triplet girls from the moment they came home from the hospital. By the time they were 16 weeks old, I had trained them to sleep twelve hours a night (sleep training for triplets takes longer due to their premature size). My sleep training method was so effective and popular with triplets that parents of twins soon came knocking, asking me to help train their babies too. Soon parents of singletons and parents of older babies came calling, often pleading with me to spare them a few nights a week since I was already booked six months or more in advance with multiples.

More than ten years and 100 families since, I am still going strong without even one baby failing to sleep through the night, whether they have cleft palates, Down syndrome, colic, or other special circumstances.

✳ My Plan ✳

How does one define "sleeping though the night" when it comes to babies? For three- to four-month-olds, some define it as "11:30 PM until 5:00 AM or 6:00 AM." That doesn't sound too bad (or actually fantastic if you are going on your tenth week of sleep deprivation) until you hear, "But as many as 50 percent [of the babies] will still require a feeding around 3:00 AM." I don't know about you, but waking up every three hours is *not* my definition of sleeping through the night! And even if you fall into the 50 percent who luck out of the 3:00 AM feeding, five to six hours a night is far short of the eight to nine hours you used to get pre-baby.

This book defines sleeping through the night as

twelve hours by twelve weeks. That means by the time your baby is twelve weeks old, she will be able to sleep from 7:00 PM to 7:00 AM (or 8:00 PM to 8:00 AM, and so on) without eating, without needing to be picked up and rocked back to sleep, without placing a lost pacifier in her mouth. In short, she will be able to sleep continuously for twelve hours, and if she does wake, she will be able to put herself back to sleep *without you*. And if your baby needs less than twelve hours of sleep, she will be able to entertain herself quietly in her crib without yelling and demanding to be removed *by you*.

My plan involves the "The Limited Crying Solution" during training. I feel this is a realistic middle ground between the "cry it out" method, which many parents cannot stomach, and the "no cry" method, which is unrealistic for many babies. For example, older babies who have already developed poor sleeping habits will usually cry some during training as they transition to better sleeping habits.

As you read this, you may be skeptical. You may be thinking this method works for some (i.e., perfect angel babies), but it will not work for *my* babies. Your friend may fill your ears with tales of not sleeping more than four hours in a row for three years, of driving around at 2:00 AM to quiet a screaming baby in the back seat, of having to sleep on the floor of the nursery while her spouse lies lonely in the king-size bed.

There are countless stories from parents regarding their difficulty in getting their children to sleep through the night. But that does not have to be *your* babies. How do I know this? Because what I have just written is true: For more than ten years, I have been training babies, from singletons to quadruplets, to sleep twelve hours a night. And not one baby has ever failed. Ever!

While there are several books on babies and sleep, this book is geared toward the mom or dad who does not have time to read a 300-page book. Whether you are a pregnant mom pulling 60-hour work weeks inside or outside the home or a sleep-deprived dad trying your best to share the all-nighters with your wife, who is recovering from a C-section, you will be able to read the key sections of this manual in *two hours*.

My promise to you is that in two hours, you will have all the tools to be able to coach your baby to sleep through the night. My book is geared toward singletons and twins. In fact, I use the terms "baby" and "babies" interchangeably throughout. The only real difference in sleep training one baby versus two or three babies, other than the number of trainees, is the timeline: You can begin training a singleton to sleep through the night earlier that multiples. Otherwise the process is the same. Any minor differences in training multiples will be discussed in separate sections entitled "Multiples."

The same goes for older babies: Although this book is aimed at training your babies to sleep through the night by twelve weeks of age, the same methods apply to training babies throughout the first year and even up to 18 months of age. In other words, if your five-month-old, nine-month-old, or twelve-month-old is keeping you up all night, it is not too late—this book can help you train your baby to sleep twelve hours a night in about one to two weeks.

Although there is some material in this book dedicated to my philosophies on why it is important for infants to sleep through the night and the consequences of them not doing so, this book is mainly a practical how-to guide. I like to think of it as being no more difficult to read through than the directions included with a bouncy seat (a device to be shunned and avoided if you use the vibration feature, but more on that later). My method is clearly laid out with easy-to-read headings and lots of practical examples. I also provide charts to help explain my method and for you to photocopy and use during training.

I am called the "Baby Coach" because that is what I do: coach babies to sleep through the night. It is similar to being a personal trainer: Parents can learn to teach their babies to sleep through the night on their own, just like parents can exercise and work out on their own. But it is a lot easier if you have someone design a program for you to follow, and encourage you along the way. That is what I hope this book will do for you and your babies: give you a step-by-step program on how to train your babies to sleep through the night.

Just because you have children does not mean you have to live in a sleep-deprived coma for three to five years. Order, structure, and sanity can be yours again. If you are willing to "coach" your babies using the methods that I outline in this book, you can save yourself months or even years of living in a state of being I describe as "just getting by," a detrimental mind-set for you and your baby. Prepare yourself: You are about to see how truly wonderful being a parent can be when you and your baby get the sleep you should.

People call me the Baby Coach. I call myself the person who has the best job in the world—I work with babies.

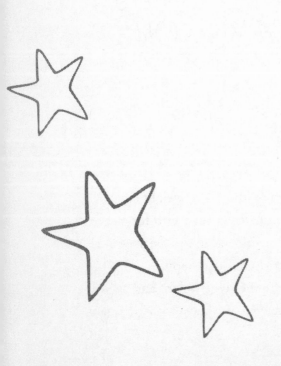

Chapter 1

The Promise of Twelve Hours' Sleep by Twelve Weeks Old

$\mathcal{L}$et's get right to it. In short, the program I teach is this:

1. Babies who are the right weight and age sleep or rest quietly in their crib for twelve hours at night, one hour in the morning, and two hours in the afternoon.

2. Babies who are the right weight and age eat four times during the day with no night

feedings. Each feeding time should last about
30 minutes.

How do you get babies to sleep twelve hours by
twelve weeks old? I believe that babies would do this on
their own if parents just left them alone and encouraged
their babies' natural tendencies. But twenty-first-
century parenting is wrought with insecurity. Web
sites, books, and talk shows now figure in along with
neighbors, friends, and family on how to raise a baby.
So many people are talking in your head—do this,
don't do this, you are not doing this right, you are not
doing that right. You don't hold your baby enough,
you hold your baby too much. An already nervous
and fearful parent can sometimes be paralyzed by all
of this well-intentioned but often conflicting advice.

And even if we are secure in our parenting skills,
lack of sleep clouds our judgment. Before you were a
mother, you were a human being who required a certain amount of sleep during each 24-hour period.

After a few weeks of sleeping two to four hours a
night, many of my clients hit a wall, and their pri-
mal need for sleep takes over their rational decision-
making skills. What happens is that you go for what I
call the "quick fix"—you know it is wrong, but you

just want the baby to stop crying, and stop crying *right now*. So what do you do? You break out the swing, put the calming vibrations on the maximum setting, or allow your baby to snack on the bottle or breast every hour, all in a desperate effort to make the baby sleep so you can sleep. The short-term fix then turns into a daily habit that you do not know how to break.

I do not make these same mistakes because sleep training is my job and I work when well rested. I have been doing this for more than ten years, so the panic and confusion that goes along with parenting, especially for the first time, is not there. I also know when the babies are naturally going to start stretching their feeding and sleeping times, and I use this to my advantage during training.

My work with a family can range from a 45-minute phone consultation to working 8–12 hours a night, seven days a week, for the first twelve weeks after the baby comes home from the hospital. Some people just communicate with me through the message board on my Web site. But no matter how much time I spend with a family, the goal is the same: to give you and your child the tools necessary to sleep twelve hours a night.

✳ Four Foundations of Baby Sleep Success ✳

1. A baby must adapt to the existing family; the existing family does not adapt to a baby.

Although some change is necessary on the part of the family, a new baby should not dictate the when, where, and how of normal family life. As simple and important as this concept is, it can be a difficult concept for first-time parents to accept. Yet babies are adaptable, and they should be exposed to all facets of family life. For example, doorbells can ring, older siblings can laugh out loud, the washing machine can run, all during naptime. Otherwise, the existing family ends up living in a fearful and tense environment in which even breathing is frowned upon. Furthermore, you have taught your baby to sleep only in a noiseless, artificial environment. Unless you are prepared to shelter your baby in the house forever, this sleeping pattern will eventually fail.

2. You must feel empowered as a parent.

It is important to say to yourself, "I am the parent, I am in charge. You are the baby, you follow my guidelines." Because without parental empowerment, an inexperienced and ill-equipped leader takes over: the baby! Parents often blame and resent the baby for problems that arise from this, mostly because they feel helpless. Instead, children need an authoritative figure, even at this young age, who will set boundaries and limits. Kids need to know that when they break the rules, the rules will be enforced. Otherwise you are placing the weight and burden of child-rearing on them, and that is not fair.

Once you are empowered by the fact that "I am the parent," you also need to realize that you cannot protect your baby from everything. You are entrusted with your child for a short period and need to help him build skills during that time. Your job is to teach your child the skills he needs so he can go out on his own and survive the best he can. A good parent is not one who has all the rules and solutions; it is one who says, "I have to get my child ready for the world." Because whatever you don't teach your child, life will, and life is not as kind.

As children grow older, you will still act as a rule enforcer, but gradually they will develop the ability to make their own decisions. As a parent, you give them the tools to make good decisions. You teach them to make their own decisions by slowly giving them more responsibility and more opportunities to make choices, as related to their age.

Another part of parental empowerment is the need to filter information in terms of what makes sense for your family. Do not feel like you have to incorporate every piece of advice on child-rearing that you hear. You, not a talk show queen, not Babythis& Babythat.com, not your Aunt Mary, are the ultimate decision maker when it comes to raising your child.

3. Sleeping is a learned skill that you need to teach your baby.

It is unbelievable what babies can learn. The babies I work with overwhelm me every single time because they never fail me. I find that babies often learn by stumbling across things and then realize, "Oh, this is how it works!" Your role as a parent is to recognize and encourage these positive discoveries.

Sleeping soundly is a basic, teachable skill. It is as necessary and important as learning how to talk, learning how to walk, and other milestones in a baby's mental and physical development. And just as you encourage your baby to talk by sounding out "M-O-M-

M-A" slowly and repeating the word over and over again, or encouraging your baby to walk by placing a toy just slightly out of reach and saying, "Come here, you can do it," you should also encourage good sleep skills by giving your baby the opportunity to self-soothe and put herself to sleep without you or other aids.

Rocking a twelve-week-old baby over and over again in a glider until he falls asleep is the equivalent of carrying a two-year-old toddler everywhere in your arms over and over again. In each case, the babies have the ability to sleep or walk, respectively, but the parents are constantly "fixing" it for them instead of guiding the babies to do it on their own.

Just as learning to walk involves some stumbling and falling along the way, learning to recognize fatigue and learning to fall and remain asleep will involve some pitfalls as well. But just as your child will eventually master the skill of walking with your guidance and encouragement, and just as you do not forget how to walk after spraining an ankle, sleeping is a skill a baby will never forget if he gets sick or goes on vacation. In fact, babies become better and better at sleeping with time.

4. Sleep training requires commitment and hard work on the part of the parents.

This foundation is pretty self-explanatory: Like most good things in life, parents will need to put some effort into sleep training. And even after training is completed, parents will need to reinforce what they have taught their children from time to time, especially when children are sick or are going through a difficult developmental stage, whether it be teething or transitioning from the crib to the "big bed."

✳ Six Benefits of Baby Sleep Success ✳

1. There is little crying involved.

I do not believe there is a lot of learning going on after five minutes of steady, continuous crying. As a result, my method is not as fast as some sleeping methods, but it works 100 percent of the time. You will not have to go through periods of listening to your baby cry continuously without interruption. I believe in The Limited Crying Solution, which limits crying to five minutes at a time. Long stretches of cold-turkey screaming might get you from point A to point B faster, but in my opinion, it can be emotionally damaging for both the parent and the child. Likewise, while some babies can be trained to sleep through the night with no crying, for many babies this is an unrealistic approach. Instead, I use small "baby" steps instead of large steps to get your baby to sleep.

Letting a baby cry all night long without doing anything to enable her to calm down goes against the natural nurturing feeling of the parents. As a result, the parents feel uncomfortable and might not stick with the training. I want parents to feel good about the sleep-training process and see results that empower them to move on.

2. You will have happier, more cooperative children.

Babies who have a schedule, sleep through the night, and have good sleeping and eating habits are happy babies. These babies always know where their place in the family is and they always know who is in charge. They know the love is there, they know the structure is there, and they know the security is there. In their little world there is no confusion, no insecurity, no not knowing. Their whole world makes sense to them.

Because they are well rested, these babies will be more alert and more willing to listen during their awake times, which in turn means they will be more active learners. They will also be more willing to play contentedly by themselves and not require constant entertainment by parents and other caregivers.

This contentment will continue to grow as they grow. They will be more approachable and more social because they do not have to have their way all the time. They will say to themselves, "I don't have to have that toy, I know how to share. I have always shared everything because I am a part of, not the center of, my family." The ability to self-console also leads to self-control, so hopefully you can avoid the two year old's screaming meltdown in the parking lot of the mall that we have all had the pleasure of witnessing at some point in our lives.

In essence, they will have a more peaceful and secure journey through toddlerhood. The structure and stability of their everyday routine will give them the "road map" to get from infancy to kindergarten without having to figure it out on their own and learn the hard way.

This is because you have laid down a foundation

for good sleeping, eating, and other skills that babies can build upon themselves once they leave the baby stage.

3. You will be using proactive parenting.

Your babies will benefit from *your* sleep as well. Instead of "just making it through" in a zombie-like, sleep-deprived state during the day, you will have the energy to proactively parent your child in terms of play and conversation with your baby.

4. You will have a predictable schedule.

If you follow my plan, you will have the luxury of knowing that for one hour in the morning, two hours in the afternoon, and three to four hours at night before your own bedtime, your time is your own. You can put your feet up and read a book, take a bath, or take your own nap because you know your baby will be sleeping or playing quietly in her crib during that time.

5. You will be able to deal with more than one child effectively.

How can you constantly tend to a baby when you have a toddler who needs attention? Or you have a new baby on the way? It is not realistic. That approach will work for only one baby. My plan will help you effectively handle multiple children, giving you the freedom to function as a family.

6. You can follow this plan on your own.

For the parents I have worked with for the full twelve weeks, many of them dread my departure once we come to the end of the twelve weeks. They believe I have some sort of magic sleep wand. But I am just an orchestrator. The true ability to sleep through the night is with the babies and the parents themselves.

The first night the babies sleep through the night and I am not there the parents think, "Oh, that was a lucky event." The second night they say, "Oh, wow, they did it again!" The third night, "They did it again?!?!?" Then the parents transition their thinking to, "Oh, the babies are sleeping through the night, maybe this is here to stay." A week goes by without me at their house, but I am still talking to the parents by phone. Then they call me only once the following week. Then the parents realize, "I haven't called Suzy in a month—I don't need Suzy anymore!" Then they say, "Suzy who?"

You can have the same experience by reading this book. I have worked with many, many families who could not afford me for seven days a week, so I would go one or two nights a week, and they trained the babies themselves on the other five to six nights. Or I consulted with them only by phone a few times. As long as you are consistent in applying what you read and truly believe in my plan for baby sleep success, it can work from a distance too.

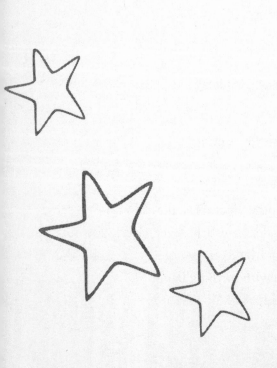

Chapter 2

Weeks 1–6

✳ Take It Easy, But Do Not Create Bad Habits ✳

For the first four to six weeks, you are off the hook as far as serious sleep training goes. I really do not start sleep training and coaching until the babies are about four to six weeks old, depending on weight, prematurity, and other factors. Take this time to let your body recover, let your babies get used to life outside the womb, and let everyone get used to all the changes that come with birthing babies.

That being said, read this chapter carefully, because you do not want to create bad habits that you will need to break later. You cannot spoil babies before twelve weeks of age, but you can create bad habits. That is because babies just follow along, and it is your job to guide them in the right direction.

Pre–sleep training is kind of like pre-dieting. If you eat a pint of Häagen-Dazs ice cream every day for eight weeks, your body is really going to have a hard time giving that up when you start the diet. If you only have that 1,200-calorie treat every three to four days, then your body is not as used to it. The ice cream is not a daily habit.

The same thing goes for a baby. If you put your baby in a swing every single time she cries for the first six weeks, she will expect you to put her in the swing each and every time she cries *after* six weeks. The baby cries, you put her in the swing. The baby cries, you put her in the swing. Over and over again, you repeat the same pattern. Soon the baby cries and she *needs* the swing. The swing changes from being one way to help the baby calm down to being the *only* way the baby can calm down. It is not her fault; the baby is just doing what you taught her to do. I personally am not a big fan of swings or the use of the vibration mode in bouncy chairs and bassinets. Using the vibration mode does all the work for your baby, so he never learns to soothe himself. I see these as quick fixes that disable an infant from learning to self-soothe, the crux of teaching your child to sleep through the night.

Pacifiers, on the other hand, are a very effective tool in helping to teach your baby to self-soothe. However, I would try to use pacifiers only while your baby is in the crib for naps and night sleep. Otherwise, you stand the chance of creating a two-and-a-half-year-old toddler running around all day with a pacifier in her mouth.

I am also not opposed to thumb-sucking: It is a form of self-soothing, and as long as your baby's thumb is not hermetically sealed to his mouth 24/7, it is a permissible habit during the baby's first year.

I would never use the swing or the vibration setting in chairs and bassinets with the intent to calm a baby or, worse still, to encourage sleep. Instead, I would use other consolation techniques in rotation to soothe a fussy baby, such as rocking her in a glider, placing her over your knee and massaging her back, or offering her a pacifier (please see Chapter 4 for a list of other possible consolation methods you can use).

That way the baby will learn that crying does not equal swing, crying does not equal being vibrated. Crying equals many different methods of consoling.

There will be times when the baby and/or you are in total meltdown crisis mode. The baby is screaming from gas pain and you are in desperate need of a bathroom break. Or you are on your fourth Luna Bar of the day and need some time to eat "real" food. It's fine to pull out the swing or the vibrating bouncy chair. Just make sure that you use these devices sparingly, almost like breaking the glass on the "use in case of emergency" fire extinguisher. Remember, use all the devices you have to help you in a crisis, but when you are not in crisis, try to stay away from them.

I do love bouncy seats when they are used without vibration. Between birth and three months, the chairs keep the babies in an upright position from which they can safely look around and take in their surroundings. This is a welcome break for young infants, who spend a great deal of time viewing the world while on their backs. In addition, the upright position helps babies keep stomach acids down and aids in the early digestion of food. As they get older, the babies will be able to rock themselves in the chair. Unlike vibrating, this is a form of self-soothing, the main theme of my method. You are creating an environment in which your baby will learn to calm himself, soothe himself, and be more comfortable by himself. These three skills are vital to baby sleep success.

✳ Create a Log ✳

In the hospital, you probably took part in charting three important events that occur in the lives of all newborns:

1) What time baby ate.
2) How much baby ate.
3) What time you changed baby's diaper and what was inside (urine or stool).

I cannot stress how important it is to continue charting these three events after your baby comes home from the hospital and until training is completed. Not only will it help you train your baby to

sleep through the night, but it will also help you recognize when your baby is sick, not eating well, and
other events. It will also help you specifically recall
what happened two days before, during a time in your
life when the days will blend together into a sleep-
deprived haze. If you have several caregivers, such as a
nanny or your husband, the log serves as an excellent
communication tool between caregivers.

I have created three 24-hour daily logs that you
can photocopy. The first starts at 12:00 AM, the second
starts at 7:00 AM, and the third starts at 8:00 AM. Please
feel free to use whichever one works best for you. Or
you may wish to use the 12:00 AM log for the first six
to eight weeks and then transition to the 7:00 AM or
8:00 AM log once you begin training.

In addition to the three events listed above, I have
added a "Notes" section. You can use this for record-
ing special events, such as your baby's first smile, or
not-so-special events, such as vomiting, diarrhea, and
other health issues, such as medications. There is also
a sample daily log sheet so you can get an idea of what
information to include.

NAME				Date	
AM	Bottle (oz.)	Breast (min.) L/R	Urine	Stool	Notes
12: ___					
1: ___					
2: ___					
3: ___					
4: ___					
5: ___					
6: ___					
7: ___					
8: ___					
9: ___					
10: ___					
11: ___					
PM					
12: ___					
1: ___					
2: ___					
3: ___					
4: ___					
5: ___					
6: ___					
7: ___					
8: ___					
9: ___					
10: ___					
11: ___					

Twelve Hours' Sleep by Twelve Weeks Old

NAME _____			Date _____		
AM	Bottle (oz.)	Breast (min.) L/R	Urine	Stool	Notes
7: ___					
8: ___					
9: ___					
10: ___					
11: ___					
PM					
12: ___					
1: ___					
2: ___					
3: ___					
4: ___					
5: ___					
6: ___					
7: ___					
8: ___					
9: ___					
10: ___					
11: ___					
AM					
12: ___					
1: ___					
2: ___					
3: ___					
4: ___					
5: ___					
6: ___					

Weeks 1–6

AM	Bottle (oz.)	Breast (min.) L/R	Urine	Stool	Notes
NAME _____			**Date** _____		
8: ___					
9: ___					
10: ___					
11: ___					
PM					
12: ___					
1: ___					
2: ___					
3: ___					
4: ___					
5: ___					
6: ___					
7: ___					
8: ___					
9: ___					
10: ___					
11: ___					
AM					
12: ___					
1: ___					
2: ___					
3: ___					
4: ___					
5: ___					
6: ___					
7: ___					

NAME 5-week-old twin					Date 07/20
AM	Bottle(oz.)	Breast(min.)L/R	Urine	Stool	Notes
7: 15		15L/10R	Full ✓	✓	Reflux medicine
8: ___					
9: ___			✓		
10: 00		10L/15R		✓	Diarrhea - watch
11: ___					
PM					
12: 45		15L/15R	✓	✓	Checked temp. 100.1
1: ___					
2: ___					
3: 45		10L/10R	✓		
4: ___					
5: ___					
6: 15		10L/10R	✓		Reflux medicine
7: ___					
8: ___					Baby extra fussy
9: 15	3.5		✓		Diaper rash cream
10: ___					
11: ___					
AM					
12: 00	4		✓	✓	Sleepy during nursing
1: ___					
2: ___					
3: 00	4		✓	✓	
4: ___					Diaper check
5: 45	3		✓	✓	
6: ___					

✳ Feedings During the Day ✳

Your babies should be able to eat every 2½–3 hours during the day for the first six weeks. Your feeding schedule during the first six weeks should mirror the babies' feeding schedule while they were in the hospital. This means two things:

1) Babies need to eat every three hours because steady weight gain is very important in the first few weeks of life.

You will need to wake up your baby to feed him if he is sleeping past the three-hour mark. In addition, you do not want your baby to get into the habit of sleeping for long stretches of five to six hours during the day. You want these stretches to occur at night.

You will spend a lot of time waking your baby in order to feed during these weeks. It is not always easy to do. A good way to rouse your baby to eat is by changing her diaper or by stroking her cheek with your finger.

✳ *EXAMPLE:* The baby's last feeding started at 10:00 AM and it is now 1:00 PM, three hours since the start of the baby's last feeding. The baby is still sleeping. You need to wake the baby up so that she is eating every three hours.

2) It is also important not to feed your baby more frequently than every two and a half hours during the first six weeks, unless there is a medical reason and your pediatrician advises you follow a more frequent feeding schedule. Your baby's digestive system needs time to process the food. Feeding every 1½–2 hours will lead your baby to snack instead of eating complete meals because there is still unprocessed food from the last feeding in his stomach. It will also make training your baby to eat on a four-hour schedule in the future more difficult.

✳ *EXAMPLE:* The baby last ate at 2:00 PM. It is now 4:00 PM and the baby is fussy. Try to help the baby not eat until at least 4:30 PM (please see the daytime toolbox in Chapter 4, which will arm you with the information and tools to get your fussy baby through the next 30 minutes to an hour without feeding).

Because your baby is still adjusting to his new environment, do not expect much interaction with him.

He will not be awake that often. However, this is the best time to indulge yourself in your babies by holding them and bonding with them while keeping a preventative eye out for bad habits.

It is important to let your baby eat as much as she wants, especially during the day. Unless your pediatrician has prescribed a more limited feeding regime, let your baby eat until she is satisfied. This will help with training later on once you move to four feedings per day. If your baby is used to feeding until she is full, her metabolism will naturally set how much she eats at each feeding.

Also, do not get caught up with how much your baby eats at any one feeding. Instead, look at how much your baby eats during a 24-hour period. As long as she taking in an adequate amount per day, whether she eats more in the morning or evening is not as pertinent.

✳ *MULTIPLES:* During the day, I strongly advise feeding your babies at the same time (tandem nursing if you are breastfeeding) or as close to the same time as possible (i.e., one right after the other) throughout all stages of training and beyond. This will not only facilitate training, but will free up more time for other activities, such as letting your babies practice their eye-movement skills by looking at a mobile or letting you make a cup of coffee, and drink it while it is still warm!

✳ Feeding During the Night ✳

Feeding your baby at night is similar to feeding your baby during the day in that you do not want to feed your baby more frequently than every two and a half hours. How long you let your baby go between feedings at night, however, depends on whether you have a singleton or twins.

For a singleton, you will need to wake your baby every three hours for a feeding *for at least the first three to four weeks*. For twins, you will need to wake your babies every three hours for a feeding for *at least the first five to six weeks*.

These steps are to ensure proper weight gain. Twins are born weighing less than singletons, usually, and therefore need more feedings for a longer period of time to catch up.

After three to four weeks for singletons and five to six weeks for twins, you can let the baby or babies start to stretch the time naturally between night feedings on their own, depending on their weight, prematurity, and other factors.

✳ Sleeping During the Night ✳

For part or all of the first six weeks, your baby will be waking up to eat every 2½–3 hours. I advise parents to develop a plan before the baby is born so that each parent can get a solid chunk of sleeping time if possible. Try to take into account your natural sleep patterns (Mom is a night owl, while Dad likes to be up at the crack of dawn) when making these plans.

> ✳ *EXAMPLE:* Mom feeds the baby between 10:00 PM and 3:00 AM while Dad sleeps. Dad feeds the baby between 3:00 AM and 8:00 AM while Mom sleeps.

Although there is no sleep training going on during the first six weeks, I would still encourage your baby just to sleep and eat at night. Do not foster wake time. Keep the lights low, feed the babies, and put them right back in their crib.

If your baby seems fussy between night meals, I would do a quick check for potential problems:

- *Is she too hot?* Check her forehead.
- *Is she too cold?* Check her nose and hands.
- *Is she spitting up?* Tilt her crib with phone books securely positioned under the two far legs of the crib or tilt the baby herself with special wedges you can buy at baby supply stores to prevent reflux and keep her stomach acids down.
- *Is she uncomfortable?* Young infants do not have a good command of their muscles and body movement, so shift them into different positions.
- *Does she have a dirty diaper?* Check to see if she has a poopy or a full wet diaper and change if necessary.

Babies should sleep in their cribs, in the nursery. While some experts think it is fine for babies to sleep in their parents' room, either in a crib or the parents' bed for the first six weeks, I disagree. The parents' bedroom is an adult safe haven. It also sets up a bad habit that the parents have a tough time breaking after the first six weeks have passed. The baby learns to depend constantly on the parents to fall and stay asleep. This is the antithesis of what my plan is about.

✳ *MULTIPLES:* Many parents prefer to have their twins and even triplets sleep in the same crib for the first few months. After all, they have already slept together for the first nine months of their lives in utero. This is fine for the first eight to nine weeks, and probably helps ease the transition to life on the outside.

But once sleep training begins in earnest, I prefer that multiples sleep in separate cribs. During training and afterward, they will have different sleep issues and sleep patterns that may affect each baby's ability to sleep continuously. At some point, usually around five to six months, depending on their prematurity, they will need to be separated due to size anyway.

Babies can sleep in the same room for as

long as the parents want them to. Many parents worry that one baby will wake the other baby with crying or other noise. I have found that as long as the babies have always had to share the same nursery, most will learn to sleep through and filter out noises made by the other baby or babies. But if they are in the same crib, they have to contend not only with noise a few inches instead of a few feet away, they also have to tackle flailing arms or legs that might wake anyone out of a sound sleep!

✳ Sleeping During the Day ✳

Before six weeks of age, your baby will be eating every 2½–3 hours, so do not worry about how much the baby sleeps or does not sleep between these feedings. The number and duration of these daytime naps will not affect sleeping at night until training begins.

Chapter 3

Weeks 6–8

✳ The Two-Week Storm ✳

About three years into my work as a baby coach, I noticed that, beginning around six weeks and lasting until eight weeks, almost all of the babies I worked with, even those who could best be described as "easy babies" or "perfect angels," went through a difficult period. They cried uncontrollably, had bad gas, struggled with intestinal cramps, or were restless between feedings. Although these periods varied in intensity, all babies struggled with similar problems.

After observing this pattern for more than ten years, my opinion is that almost all babies will have some form of colic—it is not a matter of whether your babies will get colic, but when and how severely. Typically this transition seems to occur between three to four weeks for singletons and six to eight weeks for twins. But the time also varies based on the baby's weight, prematurity, and other factors. It could be related to immune system changes or digestive system changes, but whatever the cause, babies seem to be at some sort of developmental crossroads at that point, and not a pleasant one, either.

Usually you will notice a clearly audible change in the baby's cry. It is a piercing cry, and the face becomes very red. The baby also might spit up more frequently and in greater volumes. It will scare you the first time—most parents call me frantically when it starts, so I have gotten into the habit of telling the families I work with to expect this one-to-two-week period ahead of time and prepare for it.

That way, when it happens, you are more in control of the situation, like when you know in advance about a snowstorm.

Instead of the unsettling experience of having to

ask, "What is happening?" you can say, "Oh, this is what Suzy was talking about. I knew this was coming and it is a stage that will soon go away." Since you know what is going on, you are not going to be as up-set and tense; when you are not as tense, your baby is not tense during this already difficult period.

✳ Speaking of Storms: Avoid the Snowball Effect ✳

Try to make this time as comfortable for your baby as possible, but, again, without creating too many bad habits you will later need to break. The two-week pe-riod can get very rough—your baby might not be able to relax or go to sleep because of the pain. Some ba-bies cry a lot and cry painfully. You can try remedies such as infant gas drops or gripe water to see if they work for your baby, or you can try to massage your baby gently during these times.

One of the worst habits I have observed is parents growing more and more tolerant of the crying. For example, at first the baby will cry for one to two min-utes before the parent will go in and pick the child up to console him. But soon, the parent's threshold of tolerance for crying expands, and they will wait five minutes before going in to console the baby. This tolerance keeps expanding, and pretty soon, some parents are going in after 15 minutes to pick up the baby. Unfortunately, the baby has learned that instead of crying one to two minutes, he now has to cry 15 minutes to get the same result: The parent picks up the baby. The baby then thinks, "After 15 minutes I (baby) get what I want, after 15 minutes they (parents) give in."

Some parents think the solution to this is waiting even more time, say 20 minutes, before responding to the baby: "The baby wants me to pick him up, so I am going to wait 20 minutes before I go into his room." The baby then thinks, "OK, I need to cry 20 minutes to get what I want." This is the snowball effect. Although the baby may have to cry longer and harder, the parent will still pick him up each and every time. The parent has not taught the baby that crying gets no results, the intended moral. The parent has taught the baby that, although the duration of the cry might vary, the result will not: Crying equals being picked up.

The baby is not the only one who now has a bad habit.

The parent has gotten into the equally bad habit of

always giving in, eventually always giving the baby what he wants. It is a two-way street: The baby gets used to demanding through crying, and the parent gets used to giving in because of the crying.

You can avoid this snowball effect by following my coaching methods below.

✳ Feeding During the Day ✳

By week six, your baby should eat every three hours during the day and eliminate the every-two-and-a-half-hour feedings. This transition might have already taken place. If not, just encourage your baby to wait the extra half hour by using the daytime toolbox found in Chapter 4. Since your baby is starting to consume more ounces per feeding, the baby needs more time to let the food digest.

✳ Feeding During the Night ✳

By six weeks, if you have not done so already, go ahead and ease up on the every-three-hours feeding schedule at night. Let your baby naturally wake up on his own to eat during the night.

✳ *EXAMPLE:* The baby usually eats every three hours at night. The baby is now six-and-a-half weeks old and last ate at 10:00 PM. It is now 1:00 AM and the baby is still sleeping. Let her sleep as long as she wants before feeding her, since your goal is to *nurture your baby's natural cue that she is capable of stretching the time between feedings.*

✳ Sleeping During the Night and Day ✳

Because this is such a difficult one-to-two-week period in your babies' development, do not worry about sleep training right now.

The six-to-eight-week period can be a tough time for the parents and the babies. But know that life gets better; you will soon go from sleep deprivation to sleep inspiration, and this book will help you get there!

Chapter 4

Weeks 8–12

✳ Let the Training Begin: ✳
Welcome to the BBC (Baby Boot Camp)

This is where the real work begins. For my plan to help your baby sleep for twelve hours by twelve weeks old, it is imperative that you train your baby in the following order.

✳ Chronological Order for Training ✳

Step 1: Feeding During the Day: Every four hours four times a day for twelve hours

Step 2: Feeding During the Night: Gradually eliminate all night feedings for twelve hours

Step 3: Sleeping During the Night: Sleeping or resting quietly in crib for twelve hours

Step 4: Sleeping During the Day: Sleeping or resting quietly in crib for about one hour in the morning and about two hours in the afternoon

Although it is important to follow the steps in this order, there oftentimes will be overlap between Steps 2 and 3.

✳ *EXAMPLE:* If you try to train your baby to sleep through the night *before* he is eating every four hours during the day, the training will not work as well, or will fail altogether. The same is true if you try to train your baby to do all four things at once. However, while you are eliminating night feedings (Step 2), you *should* start to establish your bedtime routine (Step 3).

✳ The Three Requirements ✳

Before you can teach your baby to sleep through the night using my plan, there are three requirements that must be met:

1: Weight: Baby must be at least nine pounds
2: Food: Baby eats at least 24 ounces of breast milk or formula in 24 hours.
3: Age: Baby must be at least four weeks old if a singleton.
Baby must be at least eight weeks old if a twin.
Baby must be at least twelve weeks old if a triplet.

Usually these three factors come together at the same time naturally, but sometimes you must wait a few more weeks for the baby to reach the nine-pound mark, especially if the baby was born before 36 weeks.

✳ Your Toolboxes ✳

Whenever you have a problem, it is always nice to have the right tools handy. If you have to fumble around to find the tools you need, not only do you waste precious time, but the problem often worsens. This is why I have developed daytime and nighttime toolboxes to use with your baby during training.

Emotionally, babies need some soothing from Mom and Dad in order to learn how to soothe themselves. Your mantra should be, "I cannot fix everything for you, but while you are learning to fix things for yourself, I will go through it with you by your side." Basically, you will walk the path toward sleeping through the night with your babies until they can walk on their own.

There are several things you can do to encourage your babies during training:

DAYTIME TOOLBOX

When the baby is awake during the day but having a tough time making it to the next feeding, the key is to DISTRACT, DISTRACT, DISTRACT:

- Offer pacifier—this is my first choice and usually buys you at least an extra 15 minutes of time.
- Place baby in a bouncy seat and entertain him with the bouncy seat music or your own toys and songs.
- Place baby on an activity mat or gym.
- Bounce baby on your knee and sing "Humpty Dumpty" or other nursery rhymes.
- Entertain baby with his favorite games and activities.

If the baby is falling asleep way before naptime, you can also use the consolation methods above, but do not offer the pacifier. This will push your little one over the edge into dreamland in no time. Remember, it is just as bad to have your baby fall asleep too early as it is for him to stay awake too long.

NIGHTTIME TOOLBOX

When the baby is in the crib, reassure him that, although you are not going to pick him up, you are right there. Stand next to the crib, or sit on a glider ottoman or chair so you are close to the baby.

- Offer pacifier.
- Pat baby's tummy with your hand or an emotional toy or blankie. (I encourage parents to use one toy or blanket as an emotional crutch. See page 100).
- Place your hand firmly on baby's tummy.
- Shush baby by making the shushing sound "Shush . . . shush . . . shush."
- Whisper things like "Everything is fine," "It's all right," "Mommy is here," "Daddy loves you," "I know it's hard to be a baby," etc.
- Turn baby around in the crib, place him on his side, etc. to help him find the most comfortable position.
- Show baby his emotional toy or blankie.
- Turn on his crib music toy.

These soothing techniques work two ways. They help the baby calm down, and they help you stay focused and relaxed so you can continue to train.

As you talk to your baby, you are actually talking to yourself, thinking, "My baby is going to be OK."

It is important to use good judgment with these

toolboxes. When using your daytime tools, for example, it is better to give in and feed your baby a few minutes before the desired feeding time if your baby is extremely frustrated or uncomfortable.

Likewise, there may be times when you need to take your baby out of the crib to calm him if all your nighttime tools have failed. However, these special exceptions should be rare tools of last resort, like the swing. If they become the rule and not the "exceptional" exception, training will take longer or fail altogether.

✴ The Three-Day Rule: ✴
Good Habits Take Three Days to Make and Three Days to Break

Day 1: Dark
Day 2: Gray
Day 3: White

In my work, I have found that it generally takes three days to make a positive habit, and three days to break it. Day 1 is always the worst, so this is the Dark day. Chances are very slim that Day 2 will be as bad as

Day 1, which is why I see this as the Gray day; it is almost always calmer. By Day 3, the baby has usually figured it out, so this is the White day. Although this may seem basic and obvious, it is important to remind yourself of this general rule while you are training so you know there is light at the end of the tunnel.

✴ The Seven-Day Rule: ✴
Bad Habits Take Three Days to Make
and SEVEN Days to Break

When breaking bad habits, I always tell my clients to prepare themselves for the worst and hope for the best, and that they will fall somewhere in the middle. Running into the nursery every morning as soon as you hear your baby make a sound is an example of a bad habit you are trying to break. It is important to be conscious of the extra time it takes to break bad habits so that you have the proper resolve and determination to fix them.

✳ Give In to Your Heart, Just Not 24/7 ✳

During training and beyond, I always tell my clients that this special early time with your babies will not come back. I advise them to give in to their hearts from time to time, just not 24/7. It is OK to have a slice of cake; one slice will not make you grow fat. Baby cuddle time is the same—do it, do not overdo it. The best time to cuddle and love your baby is when he is quiet and cooperative, not when he is crying. Otherwise you are rewarding negative behavior. I like to use the following example with my clients: Your baby is cooing contentedly in the bouncy seat, looking at his mobile. You say to yourself, "Aha, I am going to make that phone call now while the baby is quiet." While you are talking on the phone, you hear "Wah." You call to your son, "What's wrong, baby?" and he quiets down for a few more seconds. Then you hear "Wah, wah," and you walk closer to your baby to see what is the matter. Next you hear "Wah, wah, wah." At this point you hang up the phone and pick your baby up.

Of course this scenario is going to take place some of the time—crying babies need some parental comfort and soothing and you need to get things done while the baby is happy by himself. But when it becomes your regular pattern and you do not interact much with your baby when he is already content, you have taught the baby that crying equals parental attention. If you interact with your baby a fair amount when he is quiet and cooperative, you have taught a better lesson: I do not need to cry to get attention.

✳ STEP 1: ✳
Feeding During the Day

Before you can start working on the sleep schedule, you have to start with the daytime feeding schedule. What you do during the day is just as important as what you do at night. Here is Step 1:

Feed your baby every four hours four times a day.

If you consult your log, you have probably noticed a natural increase in the amount of food your baby eats at each feeding. He might have been eating 3 ounces every 2½–3 hours at four weeks, but then he starts eating 4 ounces every three hours at six weeks and on up the line. Most babies start eating more during the day and stretching the time between feedings. You are going to continue to encourage this natural tendency until your baby is eating every four hours from when he begins his day until he ends his day back in the crib.

If you have been feeding your baby about every three hours, the transition to every four hours will be easier than if you have been letting your baby eat small meals and snack every one to two hours. Here is how you can train your baby to eat every four hours during the day:

Divide your day into two twelve-hour parts.

The beginning times of these two twelve-hour blocks should be based on your family's needs, whether it is Dad's work schedule, your five year old's elementary school schedule, your desire to work out every morning before your baby wakes, or other family needs.

The illustrations that follow will usually be based on a 7:00 AM to 7:00 PM or an 8:00 AM to 8:00 PM model because these are popular with my clients and are easier to understand than 6:45 AM to 6:45 PM or 7:30 AM to 7:30 PM. But feel free to use blocks based on the quarter hour, half hour, or whatever works best for your family. Keep in mind that most babies seem to favor bedtimes between 7:00 PM and 9:00 PM.

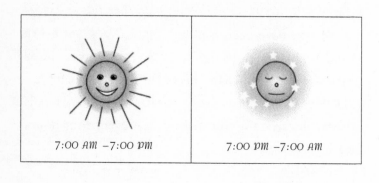

7:00 AM –7:00 PM   7:00 PM –7:00 AM

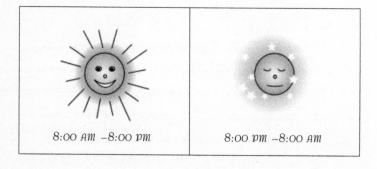

8:00 AM –8:00 PM   8:00 PM –8:00 AM

✻ *EXAMPLE:* The first part can be 6:00 AM to 6:00 PM and the second part can be 6:00 PM to 6:00 AM. You can also use 7:00 AM to 7:00 PM, 8:30 AM to 8:30 PM, or even 11:00 AM to 11:00 PM. My clients who were musicians in bands that played at night used the 11:00 AM to 11:00 PM blocks. Remember, the baby should adapt to fit into the existing family; the family should not make changes to conform to the baby's life.

Create four feeding times that are four hours apart during the day

✳ *EXAMPLE*: If your first twelve-hour block begins at 7:00 AM, then 7:00 AM + 4 hours = 11:00 AM, 11:00 AM + 4 hours = 3:00 PM, 3:00 PM + 4 hours = 7:00 PM. Thus your first feeding is at 7:00 AM, your second feeding is at 11:00 AM, your third feeding is at 3:00 PM, and your fourth and final feeding is at 7:00 PM.

First Feeding	Second Feeding	Third Feeding	Fourth Feeding
7:00 AM	11:00 AM	3:00 PM	7:00 PM

✳ *EXAMPLE*: If your first twelve-hour block begins at 8:00 AM, then 8:00 AM + 4 hours =

12:00 PM, 12:00 PM + 4 hours = 4:00 PM, and
4:00 PM + 4 hours = 8:00 PM. Thus your first
feeding is at 8:00 AM, your second feeding is at
12:00 PM, your third feeding is at 4:00 PM, and
your fourth and final feeding is at 8:00 PM.

First Feeding	Second Feeding	Third Feeding	Fourth Feeding
8:00 AM	12:00 PM	4:00 PM	8:00 PM

Feed baby at the beginning of each four-hour block

The First Feeding

Start feeding the baby at the beginning of the first
four-hour block. That means the baby wakes up or
you take her out of her crib about 15 minutes before
the first feeding time, change her diaper, dress her, and
begin feeding.

✳ *EXAMPLE:* The baby's first feeding time is
set for 8:00 AM. At around 7:45 AM, take the
baby out of the crib to be diapered and dressed,
and begin feeding her at about 8:00 AM. If you
start to get ready at 8:00 AM, you may find that
by the time you are ready to start feeding, it is

already between 8:15 AM and 8:30 AM instead of closer to 8:00 AM.

The first few days you do this, you may have to help your baby make it to the time you set for the first feeding.

Baby wakes within one hour of the first feeding time

✳ *EXAMPLE:* Baby wakes between 7:00 AM and 8:00 AM. The first feeding is at 8:00 AM.

DAY 1: The baby may wake at 7:15 AM and want to eat. The baby is not supposed to start her first feeding until 8:00 AM because she went down to sleep at 8:00 PM. Instead of feeding her as soon as she wakes, try encouraging her to last longer by using the tools in your night toolbox, such as shushing, patting her tummy, or otherwise calming her for another 15–30 minutes, until 7:30 AM, or 7:45 AM if you can.

DAY 2 and DAY 3: On Day 2, try to wait another 15–30 minutes longer than you did on Day 1. Repeat this process every morning until you reach 8:00 AM.

There might be a day or two on which you make no progress (i.e. the baby needs to eat at 7:30 AM two days in a row), or you might even go backward slightly, but if you keep pushing your baby forward to the target start time (8:00 AM in this example), you will eventually get your baby to start eating at the beginning of the first block.

The number of days your baby takes to get to the target start time is not crucial. Sometimes you have to take one step back to take two steps forward. What is crucial is that you are consistent and stick with it. Training your baby is like a diet—if you are willing to do the work, you will see results. If you cheat, you will not.

* EXAMPLE: On Day 3, you may be tempted to feed the baby at 7:15 AM instead of helping the baby make it to 7:45 AM because you want to go back to sleep.

You must fight your urge to take the easy route and use a quick fix, or else you may not get the results you want: a full twelve hours a night without having to tend to your baby for years to come.

Baby wakes up more than an hour
before the first feeding time

If your baby wakes and wants to eat and it is more than an hour before the target feeding time, it is OK to give the baby 1–2 ounces, but *only* 1–2 ounces. You should still feed the baby at the target start time as well. Just remember that over the next few days you will want to help the baby stretch the time between the snack feeding and the desired first feeding until the snack feeding is eliminated.

✳ *EXAMPLE:* Baby wakes between 6:00 AM and 7:00 AM. The first feeding is at 8:00 AM.

DAY 1: The baby wakes at 6:15 AM and wants to eat. The baby is supposed to start the first feeding of the day at 8:00 AM. Go ahead and give the baby 1–2 ounces of food at 6:15 AM and then place him back in his crib until 7:45 AM, when you begin the baby's morning routine. Then, feed him as much as he will eat at 8:00 AM.

DAY 2: The baby wakes at 6:15 AM again and wants to eat. Encourage the baby to stretch until 6:30 AM or 6:45 AM before offering 1–2 ounces.

DAY 3 and Beyond: Continue to stretch this time until you reach 7:00 AM, one hour before your scheduled feeding. Once the baby is waking to be fed around 7:00 AM, eliminate the 1–2 ounce snack feeding and follow the guidelines above to help the baby stretch his first feeding time from 7:00 AM to 8:00 AM.

Your baby is going to take baby steps to get to the first feeding time. As with learning to walk, you are going to encourage and help him along the way. I feel that my plan is a positive one: I believe in small victories, with which the baby makes steady progress during training.

The Second, Third, and Fourth Feedings During the Day

In addition to training your baby to start eating at a set time every day, you want to simultaneously encourage your baby to build up to eating every four hours throughout the day, at the start of each of your three remaining feeding times. You want to always feed your baby four hours after the *start* of each feeding, not four hours after she finishes eating.

> ✳ *EXAMPLE:* If your start time is 8:00 AM, you want to start the second feeding of the day at around 12:00 PM, the third feeding at around 4:00 PM, and the fourth and final feeding at around 8:00 PM. Whether the baby finished the third feeding at 4:15 PM or 4:30 PM is irrelevant; you will always use the 4:00 PM start time of the third feeding as your guide.

Like the first feeding, it may take a few days for your baby to go from eating every three hours to eating every four hours at the second, third, and fourth feedings. Again, take baby steps and use your daytime toolbox to help your baby slowly stretch the time between these feedings.

> ✳ *EXAMPLE: DAY 1:* Your baby's first feeding was at 7:00 AM and the second feeding is at

11:00 AM. However, it is 10:00 AM and your baby is crying and starting to root. Use the tools in your daytime toolbox, like bouncing the baby on your knee or offering a pacifier, to see if she can wait until 10:15 AM or 10:30 AM to eat.

DAY 2 and DAY 3: Help the baby wait an additional 15–30 minutes, until 10:30 AM or 10:45 AM. Repeat the process until the baby is eating at around 11:00 AM.

You will find that the second, third, and fourth feedings will all build upon each other, creating a domino effect. The longer your baby can wait between feedings, the hungrier she will be. This hunger will lead to the baby consuming more ounces, which will take longer to digest, which will in turn make it easier for your baby to stretch the time between subsequent feedings. In simpler terms, two things happen when you eliminate feedings:

1) The baby stretches the time between the four feedings.

2) The baby increases the amount she eats at each of the four feedings.

✳ *EXAMPLE:* Your first feeding was at 7:00 AM. Your baby was able to stretch her second feeding time from 10:00 AM to 10:30 AM and go from 3–3½ hours between the first feeding and the second feeding. Instead of eating her typical 3 ounces or nursing for six minutes at 10:00 AM, your baby ate 4 ounces or nursed for eight minutes at 10:30 AM. Because your baby ate 1 ounce more than usual, she should be able to stretch the time between the second and third feeding with greater ease.

I use 15-minute increments as an illustrative example for purposes of explaining my plan. If your baby can take a 20- or 30-minute step, that is fine. Your baby may need a 10-minute step once in a while, but at least 15 minutes would be my goal. But remember, every minute is a step forward toward the structure you desire.

*Once baby makes it to four hours between feedings stop
stretching the time between feedings*

✳ EXAMPLE: The second feeding began at
11:00 AM. If your baby is still sleeping at
3:00 PM, the start time of the third feeding, turn
on lights, turn on music, and otherwise make it
inviting for the baby to be awake and then feed
him. If necessary, wake your baby by 3:30 PM
and feed him. Encourage your baby to eat as
much as he can, but do not worry if he consumes less than usual. The baby might not be
as hungry at first, but he will soon adapt.

Be aware that I am not encouraging hyper-
scheduling. If you feel pressured to start feeding at exactly 3:00 PM and 15 seconds every day, you will be as
stressed as you were during the first few weeks when
your days were less predictable. I believe in a certain
amount of flexibility, in that it is fine to start feeding
5–15 minutes before or 5–15 minutes after your set
feeding times as needed.

You may notice that during the transition from
feeding every three hours or so to feeding every four

hours at scheduled times, your baby may not be eating as much. Soon he will start adding more ounces at each of the four feedings as discussed above. Remember, you are not reducing the amount of food your baby eats in a 24-hour period; you are merely concentrating the same amount of food into a lower number of feedings per day.

✳ *EXAMPLE:* Instead of eight feedings of 3–4 ounces each, you will have four feedings of 6–8 ounces each. Either way, the baby is eating 24 ounces in a 24-hour period.

As stated above, the baby should be eating at least 24 ounces in a 24-hour period before you begin training. Some babies might eat the same amount at each feeding (7 ounces at all four feedings or 18 minutes breastfeeding at all four feedings), while other babies might eat more at one feeding (i.e., 8 ounces at the first feeding, 20 minutes breastfeeding at the first feeding) and less at another (5 ounces at the second feeding, 15 minutes breastfeeding at the second feeding).

Either way is fine. What is important is that the baby consumes at least 24 ounces each day and that you let the baby eat as much as he wants at each feeding. If bottle feeding, I often recommend that you include 1–2 extra ounces in each bottle in case the baby drinks more. And if your baby is not eating as much as she should, consult your log to see when your baby naturally eats more. Then try to encourage him to eat an extra ounce or two or nurse longer at these times.

If your baby spits up some food, do not worry. It is normal for many babies to spit up some food during or after each feeding. Do not feel compelled to replace this food right there and then. The baby might be spitting up the food because she is already full. She can make up whatever amount she lost at a subsequent feeding. Besides, the amount of spit-up food oftentimes looks much greater than it actually is.

Let's say you last fed your baby at 2:00 PM, and it is now 2:45 PM and she is fussy and inconsolable. Should you feed her now or try to wait as long as possible until the next feeding? Feeding her now is better than waiting but still not making it to the next feeding time. If the baby is hungry within an hour of your last feeding time, it is OK to give the baby more food if you feel it is *truly* necessary. It is much worse to wait, say, two hours and then feed her more. Always try to stay with every four hours, especially once training is completed. And if you fail to do that, your goal for the next feeding should not be three hours, but three and a quarter, three and a half, etc. You always should stretch the baby back to the four-hour feeding times.

One question I am asked all the time is, How long should each feeding last? Ideally, during the first nine months, it should take you no more than 30 minutes to feed your baby or babies — burps, breaks, and diaper changes included.

During training, especially if you are breast- and bottle feeding simultaneously because your milk supply is low or if you are simultaneously feeding multiples, it might take you 45 minutes, but your goal should always be 30 minutes or less. Otherwise, if you take one to two hours to feed the babies, you are going to have just another two hours until you start over again. You will be feeding babies all day long.

Daytime activity

To facilitate training, make it inviting for your baby to be awake during the day, especially after each feeding. If you have been cooped up in the nursery during the first eight weeks, now is the time to take the baby to a different place in the house during the day, say, the family room, playroom, or kitchen. Be sure to return the baby to the nursery for her naps (see Step 4). This will help the baby differentiate between the sleeping/resting place (nursery) and the awake/play areas (generally the main floor of the house).

As your baby progresses through training, she will be awake for longer periods of time during the day. The baby should use these short periods of time to start playing and learning about her environment.

Here is a list of things you can do with your baby:

- Floor time (activity gym)
- Tummy time (try to wait at least a half hour to one hour after eating before tummy time. Otherwise the baby might spit up some food.)

- Massage time (best before naps or bedtime)
- Sing-along time with dancing
- Bouncy seat time
- Playpen time
- Outside time (stroller, bouncy seat, blanket under tree with toys)

Once you have your baby on a four-hour feeding schedule, try to keep your baby awake between the third and fourth feedings of the day.

This should be your baby's most active time. If the baby sleeps too much between the third and fourth feedings, she will have a difficult time going to sleep for the night after the fourth feeding.

The duration and number of naps at this time will vary. In general, your baby will take a shorter nap between the first and second feedings and a longer nap between the second and third feedings. As long as you try to keep your baby awake as best you can between the third and fourth feedings, you are on the right track.

✳ STEP 2: ✳
Feedings During the Night:
Gradually Eliminate All Night Feedings

Step 1 helps you set up the night feedings, or the lack of night feedings, and Step 2's success depends a lot on how well your days are going. Step 2's main focus is the following:

Lengthen the time between night feedings

Unlike Step 1, in which the goal is to have your baby eat every four hours during the day like clockwork, the goal at night is to have your baby go from the last feeding of the day until the first feeding of the day, twelve hours, without a feeding.

When in training during the next few weeks, feed the baby at his fourth and final day feeding, and then let him go as long as he can before the first night feeding.

This means do not wake him up for a feeding.

After this first night feeding, again, let the baby go as long as he can before the second night feeding. Repeat the process if a third night feeding exists.

Your baby might wake to feed only once or your

baby might fall into a two-feeding-per-night or three-feeding-per-night pattern. Although most of the examples that follow are based on a three-feeding-per-night pattern, these are just examples. The important thing is to work with *your* baby's pattern. So if your baby wakes to feed only once per night, that is the only feeding you have to eliminate—do not feed him two or three times per night. And you should try hard not to feed your baby more than three times per night unless medically necessary.

When the baby wakes to eat, try to minimize all stimulation. Your goal is to feed, burp, and place the baby back in the crib without fully waking him. You basically want him to sleepwalk through the night feedings: He awakens enough to eat, but ideally his eyes are closed and his movements are minimal.

Here are some tips on helping to keep the baby in a slumber-like state during night feedings:

- Do not change diaper unless it contains poop.
- Keep the room as dark as possible.
- Do not talk or make eye contact with baby (more on this topic in Step 3).
- BE PREPARED! Have your food ready to go.

Breastfeeding: Wear easy-to-access clothing.

Pumped breast milk: Serve it room temperature or place it in the warmer as soon as the baby begins to stir.

Formula: Have the water already measured in the bottle (room temperature or heating on low in the warmer) and the powder pre-measured in another container. Mix together right before you feed baby.

One of the biggest mistakes I see parents make during training is not having the bottle ready to pop into their baby's mouth during night feedings. The extra five minutes it takes to make and/or warm a bottle may seem insignificant, but in that time your baby might go from stirring and fussing to screaming with eyes wide open.

After three or four nights, you will see a definite night pattern emerge. Your log will be helpful in figuring out this pattern. The baby will tend to eat at the same times each night, just as he does during the day.

Once your baby has set her own pattern at night, you will want to let your baby "spring forward," but not "fall back": The baby can reset the clock forward but not backward.

That means it is OK for the baby to stretch beyond her regular feeding time. The time she stretches to will then become your new feeding time.

✳ *EXAMPLE:* Your baby's second night feeding was at 2:00 AM the night before, on Sunday night. It is now 2:00 AM on Monday night and your baby is still sleeping. Do not wake her to eat. Let her go as long as she can. Let's say she wakes to eat at 3:00 AM instead of 2:00 AM. Three AM becomes your new feeding time on Tuesday night.

Be prepared for her third night feeding stretching forward as well (i.e., the baby eats at 6:00 AM instead of at 5:00 AM).

It also means to try not to let the baby reset a night feeding in the opposite direction: If she wakes to feed too early, use your nighttime toolbox to help her eat at the same time she ate the night before.

However, you want to be more flexible at night than you would be during the day in order to keep your baby in a sleepwalking state: If you see your baby's milder fussing escalating to full-blown sobbing, go ahead and give her the bottle or breast earlier than scheduled.

✳ *EXAMPLE:* Your baby starts to stir at 1:30 AM, a half hour before her regular night feeding at 2:00 AM. Try to encourage her to continue to sleep by placing the pacifier in her mouth, shushing her, etc. to help her eat closer to 2:00 AM. However, if you can see that her movements and crying are growing in intensity, go ahead and feed the baby earlier. Usually she will stretch this feeding forward again during the next few days.

If you let her get to the point where arms are flying and mouth is screaming, it will be harder for her to fall asleep again after she is done eating. Remember, these nighttime feedings should enable your baby to go right back into a deep, restful sleep.

Many parents ask if you have to let the baby set the schedule at night, or if it is OK to alter it to fit the parents' sleeping needs.

I find that you get much better and faster results if you try to follow the baby's natural feeding patterns during night-weaning than if you try to establish a feeding pattern for the baby yourself.

However, you can somewhat alter the night feedings once a pattern has been established if it is more convenient for you in terms of your own continuous sleep. Be aware that you will be trading better training for convenience, however.

✳ *EXAMPLE:* The baby eats at 7:00 AM, 11:00 AM, 3:00 PM, and 7:00 PM during the day. For three to four nights in a row, you notice that he has woken up on his own around 10:00 PM, 1:00 AM, and 4:00 AM to eat. Try to follow this natural pattern when weaning the baby at night. But it is more convenient for you to feed the baby at 12:00 AM as opposed to when he might naturally awaken at 1:00 AM. It is OK to feed the baby at midnight as a reinforcement so that you can get a solid chunk of sleep yourself. Training will take a few days to a few weeks longer, though, because you are not following the baby's natural feeding schedule and you are not letting the baby "spring forward."

✳ *MULTIPLES:* When training multiples, let each baby set his own pattern. That means if one baby eats at 11:00 PM, 1:00 AM, and 5:00 AM, while the other eats at 12:00 AM, 3:00 AM, and

6:00 AM, then that is the schedule I would use during training. Remember, multiples are composed of individuals with different patterns and training issues. If you push one to eat earlier, or slow down another to eat later, training will take longer. Besides, these are temporary feedings that will disappear altogether in one to two weeks. Think of it like investing for the future— a couple of weeks of hard work and sacrificing sleep will yield tremendous dividends in terms of future sleep for many years to come. If you do the math, I think you will find that it is definitely worthwhile. That said, you can also alter your multiples' schedule to fit your own sleeping needs, as discussed in the last example.

Gradually reduce food at each night feeding, one feeding at a time.

After the baby has naturally settled into his own night pattern, you want to gradually reduce the amount of food the baby eats at each night feeding. Tackle one feeding at a time. That means you, *the parent*, should not try to reduce the amount of food for all night feedings simultaneously. But if the *baby himself* reduces the amount of food for any or all night feedings, that is fine. Once the baby eats less on his own, do not increase the amount of food for that night feeding.

✻ *EXAMPLE:* On Sunday night, the baby eats 3 ounces at the first night feeding, 2 ounces at the second night feeding, and 3 ounces at the third night feeding. On Monday night, the baby, on his own, eats 2 ounces at the first night feeding, 2 ounces at the second night feeding and 2 ounces at the third night feeding. On Tuesday night, offer the baby only 2 ounces at all three night feedings.

In my work, I have found that the baby will usually eat the least amount of food at the second night feeding so the second night feeding is usually the first to be eliminated. Then, gradually eliminate the first night feeding, and finally, eliminate the third night feeding.

Eliminate Night Feedings In This Order	Second, First, Third

To eliminate the second night feeding, you will first need to figure out the number of ounces to give your baby. This will be your starting point. Consult your log. Look at what your baby ate the night before at the second night feeding and then reduce that amount by ½ ounce.

✳ *EXAMPLE:* You are starting to reduce the amount your baby eats at the second night feeding on Monday night. On Sunday night, the baby drank 3 ounces at the second night feeding. On Monday night, I would start with 2½ ounces as your starting point since that is ½ ounce less than what the baby ate on Sunday night.

Second Night Feeding	Sun	Mon
	3 oz.	2.5 oz.

Give the baby the amount of food determined using the plan for three days in a row. Then reduce this amount by ½ ounce on Day 4.

However, if the baby drinks less than the starting point during the three days, that is your new starting point. Again, use this new starting point for three days before you reduce it by ½ ounce on Day 4 or the baby drinks less on his own.

✷ *EXAMPLE:* When the baby wakes up for
the second night feeding on Monday, give him
only 2½ ounces, the starting point determined
in our example above. You will also give
2½ ounces on Tuesday night, and 2½ ounces
on Wednesday night, for the second feeding. On
Thursday night, you will reduce the amount
of the second night feeding to 2 ounces, and
the three-day clock starts all over again. You
will keep reducing the amount of the second
night feeding by ½ ounce every four days until
the feeding is eliminated. This should take two
and a half weeks at most.

Sun.	Mon.	Tue.	Wed.	Thu.	Fri.	Sat.
3 oz.	2.5 oz.	2.5 oz.	2.5 oz.	2 oz.	2 oz.	2 oz.

Sun.	Mon.	Tue.	Wed.	Thu.	Fri.	Sat.
1.5 oz.	1.5 oz.	1.5 oz.	1 oz.	1 oz.	1 oz.	.5 oz.

Sun.	Mon.	Tue.	Wed.	Thu.	Fri.	Sat.
.5 oz.	.5 oz.	0				

However, if during those first three nights, the
baby eats less than 2½ ounces at the second night
feeding, let's say, 1½ ounces on Tuesday night, then

you will offer the baby only 1½ ounces on Wednesday night and 1½ ounces on Thursday night.

Sun.	Mon.	Tue.	Wed.	Thu.	Fri.	Sat.
3 oz.	2.5 oz.	1.5 oz.	1.5 oz.	1.5 oz.	1 oz.	1 oz.

Sun.	Mon.	Tue.	Wed.	Thu.	Fri.	Sat.
1 oz.	.5 oz.	.5 oz.	.5 oz.	0		

Be prepared for the baby to again reduce the amount offered at the second night feeding on his own, such as by eating ½ ounce on Thursday night.

Sun.	Mon.	Tue.	Wed.	Thu.	Fri.	Sat.
3 oz.	2.5 oz.	1.5 oz.	1.5 oz.	.5 oz.	.5 oz.	.5 oz.

Continue to reduce the amount of food at the second night feeding until the second night feeding is eliminated.

Once the second night feeding is eliminated, eliminate the first night feeding using the steps outlined above.

The same goes for when you eliminate the third night feeding.

Here is an example of what the first week might look like while you are eliminating the second night feeding:

Night Feeding	Sun	Mon	Tue	Wed	Thu	Fri	Sat	Sun
First	11:00 PM / 3 oz.	11:00 PM / 3 oz.	11:00 PM / 2.5 oz.	11:30 PM / 2.5 oz.	11:30 PM / 2.5 oz.	12:00 AM / 2.5 oz.	12:00 AM / 2.5 oz.	12:00 AM / 2.5 oz.
Second	1:00 AM / 2 oz.	2:00 AM / 1.5 oz.	2:00 AM / 1.5 oz.	2:00 AM / 1 oz.	2:30 AM / 1 oz.	3:00 AM / 1 oz.	3:00 AM / 0.5 oz.	0 / 0
Third	5:00 AM / 2 oz.	5:30 AM / 2 oz.	6:00 AM / 2 oz.	6:00 AM / 1.5 oz.	6:00 AM / 1.5 oz.	6:30 AM / 1 oz.	6:30 AM / 1 oz.	6:30 AM / 1 oz.

✳ *EXAMPLE:* On Sunday night, the baby ate 2 ounces at the second night feeding, so you would start to eliminate this feeding by offering 1½ ounces (½ ounce less) on Monday night. You plan to offer 1½ ounces on Tuesday and Wednesday nights but the baby on his own drinks only 1 ounce on Wednesday night. Therefore, you offer 1 ounce on Thursday and Friday nights. Since the baby did not reduce this amount on his own during the three days, you, the parent, reduce the amount on Saturday night to ½ ounce (½ ounce less than the baby drank on Friday night). You plan to offer

½ ounce on Sunday and Monday nights, but the baby does not eat anything at the second night feeding on Sunday night. At this point, the second night feeding is eliminated. Do not feed the baby any food between the first and third night feedings from now on.

Note that although you, the parent, are only reducing the food given at the second night feeding, the amount of food given at the first and third night feedings is decreasing as well. That is because the *baby on his own* is eating less at these feedings. Remember, once the baby himself eats less at any of the feedings, that is the amount you offer him from then on.

You may also note that the times for all three night feedings are moving forward, not backward. That is because you are allowing the baby himself to "spring forward," but not "fall back," as discussed.

Remember that this is only an example. Your baby may take fewer days or more days to eliminate a night feeding.

It is very important to remember two things while training the babies to eat smaller amounts and less often at night:

1. Make sure the babies are getting in those lost night ounces during the day.

Encourage the babies to eat at least an extra ½ ounce at each day feeding. Or look at what time of day they are hungriest, perhaps first thing in the morning, and try to fit an extra 1–2 ounces in at that time. The babies will naturally start to eat more during the day on their own, so it will not be a struggle to get in those extra ounces during the day.

2. Do not go backward!

Once you start training at night, try very hard not to start the night feedings too early or increase the amount of food given at any time. Progress, not regress, is your goal. Remember your mantra for these four weeks is BBC! BBC!

The hardest part about this step is often a psychological one. Twelve hours seems like a long time for your baby to go without eating. Many mothers ask me if they should supplement the last feeding of the day with rice cereal. The truth is, you don't have to. Your baby is getting enough nutrition through the feedings above.

While it is not necessary to supplement your baby's last bottle of the day with rice cereal, I do think it helps with reflux and spitting up and helps the baby more easily stretch overnight without a feeding. I would use *at most* one or two tablespoons of cereal per 6–8 ounce bottle. You are dealing with delicate digestive systems, and more than two tablespoons per bottle might create more problems than it would solve. Do not engage in faulty logic: A tablespoon of cereal does not equal an extra hour of sleep! So giving four tablespoons of cereal will not make your baby sleep four hours longer; it will probably make your baby sleep less and create a lot of laundry if your baby needs to expel the excess food.

✳ *MULTIPLES:* Again, treat the babies as individuals—reduce the amount of food at the night feeding to be eliminated based on what each baby consumes. That means if one baby eats 3 ounces at the second night feeding while the other baby eats 2 ounces at the second night feeding, you will start by giving the first baby 2½ ounces and the second baby 1½ ounces. It is the same process, but based on each baby's individual feeding pattern. Parents of multiples have more work, but they have to play the hand they were dealt. To do otherwise would not only delay training, but would be unfair to the babies.

Breastfeeding and the Elimination of Night Feedings

Clients who exclusively breastfeed their babies often ask how to gradually reduce the amount of food at each night feeding. I prefer that my clients use pumped breast milk during training for two reasons: One, you can accurately measure the amount of food your baby is getting at each feeding, and two, your baby is less likely to fall into the pattern of using the breast as a nighttime pacifier (see Chapter 6 on Extreme Circumstances).

However, if you choose to feed your baby from your breasts, apply the same reduction principles described above, but replace ounces with minutes. Just reduce the time you are feeding by three minutes every four days at the night feeding you are eliminating. If the baby nurses for a shorter period of time during any of the three days, then only let the baby nurse for this new shorter time for three days in a row, unless the baby reduces this time again on her own.

    ✳ *EXAMPLE:* If your baby nursed for 12 minutes on Sunday night at the second night feeding, let the baby nurse for 9 minutes on Monday, Tuesday, and Wednesday nights at the second night feeding.

    On Thursday night, again, reduce the time by three minutes. The baby will then nurse for six minutes on Thursday, Friday, and Saturday nights.

Sun.	Mon.	Tue.	Wed.	Thu.	Fri.	Sat.
12 min.	9 min.	9 min.	9 min.	6 min.	6 min.	6 min.

Sun.	Mon.	Tue.	Wed.	Thu.	Fri.	Sat.
3 min.	3 min.	3 min.	0 min.			

But if the baby nurses for only seven minutes on Tuesday night, then let the baby nurse for only seven minutes on Wednesday and Thursday nights as well, unless the baby again nurses for less time on her own, i.e., for five minutes on Thursday night.

Sun.	Mon.	Tue.	Wed.	Thu.	Fri.	Sat.
12 min.	9 min.	7 min.	7 min.	5 min.	5 min.	5 min.

Sun.	Mon.	Tue.	Wed.	Thu.	Fri.	Sat.
2 min.	2 min.	2 min.	0 min.			

Also record how many minutes your baby nurses at the other night feedings. If on her own she nurses for less time at those feedings, then on future nights do not let her nurse for more time at those feedings.

Make sure that you use a *digital clock* to time your feedings: It is more precise and much easier to read in the dark than an analog clock.

Breastfeeding mothers have certain issues that come up when reducing the night feedings. One of my clients told me she was afraid to stop feeding at night because she worried her milk supply would diminish. She wanted to know how to keep her milk supply consistent during training and beyond.

Since her body had been producing milk every three hours for one to two months, I told her to gradually increase the amount of time she nursed at all four day feedings by two to three minutes.

You can also pump after each day feeding for a couple of weeks to help train your body to produce more milk at these times. If you like, you can also pump before bed to maintain adequate milk production. That way, you have extra milk on hand during night training or to store for future use.

If you are nursing, I would pump only when your breasts feel full once you go to sleep for the night, full enough that they are bothersome or wake you up. I would also pump just enough to relieve the pressure (i.e., do not empty your breasts). Eventually, your body will adjust, probably in a couple of weeks.

I have found that whatever you set yourself up for, your body will follow in its own milk production rhythm. Just as your milk supply adjusts to your baby's demand, your body will adjust to your demand, letting you produce more milk during the day and less at night. You will find you can sleep longer and longer without needing to pump.

And you will produce more milk during the day because that is when your baby sucks with the greatest intensity, and your body "learns" this. Nature is unbelievable!

✳ STEP 3: ✳

Sleeping During the Night: Baby Sleeps or Has Quiet Time in Crib for Twelve Hours a Night

Establish a bedtime routine.

Thirty minutes before your fourth and final feeding of the day, take your baby up to the nursery. You will then need to do five or six things consistently each night to signal to your baby that it is time to wind down and go to sleep.

It is important to be consistent in your nighttime routine. Think about something you always do, like drink coffee, take a shower, or brush your teeth every morning. The day just doesn't go right unless you do it; something is off. Babies feel the same way.

Here is a list of nighttime rituals I recommend:

- Lower the ceiling light with a dimmer switch or turn on one or two lamps or night-lights with low-wattage lightbulbs (15 or 25 watts).
- Close the blinds or lower the shades on any windows in the nursery (I recommend

using room-darkening shades so that as you go from winter to summer or experience fall and spring time changes, your baby is not confused by the longer periods of daylight).

- Turn the radio to a soothing music station (classical, jazz, love songs) or play a lullaby or other soft-music CD.
- Give baby a bath and/or massage.
- Put on a nighttime diaper and nighttime clothes (footed sleeper, sleep sack, etc.). Nighttime diapers are important because you want to change the baby's diaper only if she has pooped. Changing wet diapers all night will interrupt sleep for both you and the baby. Change your baby into nighttime clothes, even if you do not give the baby a bath. Changing clothes in the morning and night helps the baby distinguish between night and day.
- Read to baby.
- Shut the nursery door to keep out other light and noise.

Feed baby. Use Step 2 instructions to ensure your baby is getting enough food before bedtime.

Place baby in the crib AWAKE.

The linchpin of Step 3 is that you have to put the baby in the crib while she is still awake. This is because the baby has to learn to put herself to sleep in order to be able to sleep through the night. After the baby has learned to fall asleep in the crib on her own for at least six weeks, it is fine to have her fall asleep in your arms one or two times per week, but not two nights in a row. Otherwise, the baby could develop the habit of falling asleep outside the crib and then not be able to fall asleep on her own in the crib.

Turn on a soothing musical crib toy.

This toy can be a mobile, a soft toy, or a crib soother such as the Fisher-Price Ocean Wonders Aquarium, but just make sure it plays soft, soothing music for at least 3–10 minutes. This is not the time or place for Tickle Me Elmo.

Give baby a safe, age-appropriate blankie or emotional toy that has the mother's scent.

Make sure that whatever you give your child is not a SIDS or choking risk. Before you give this toy to your baby for the first time, you should sleep with it for three to four days so it absorbs your scent. When the baby wakes up at night, she can then draw this toy close to her and be soothed by your smell without you actually being there.

Kiss baby and tell her good night.

My favorite part of Step 3.

Darken the room, leave the room, and close the door behind you.

Yes, I said to close the door. At night, you want to create a quiet sleep oasis for your baby to rest in. Make sure the room is dark enough for your baby to sleep, but use your personal preference. Some parents like it pitch-black dark because they find night-lights wake the baby throughout the night. Some parents like a small night-light or two. You will also want to use a baby monitor to check on your baby until you feel secure in your baby's sleep habits.

✷ *MULTIPLES:* If you have twins or triplets, you may need to start your bedtime routine 45–60 minutes before the fourth feeding. Try to place your babies in their cribs at the same time or within 15 minutes or so of each other.

How to Tackle Crying: The Limited Crying Solution

When people hear a baby cry, they say, "Oh my god, something must be wrong. This small and helpless baby is in distress and I need to fix it."

But sometimes the baby is just trying to talk to you.

While there are some things you can fix, such as a poopy diaper or giving him a warm blanket to sleep with, there are other things you cannot or, more accurately, should not fix.

As discussed above, crying babies do need some parental soothing. But your role should be to assist, not solve, your babies' emotional problems. Remember, your mantra should be "I cannot fix it for you, but I will go through it with you by your side." Soon, your babies will need less and less assistance because they will learn how to soothe themselves on their own.

Let baby cry three to five minutes before going into the nursery.

As hard as this step is for parents to do, it is absolutely essential to helping your baby learn to sleep through the night. As he is crying, the baby is trying to figure it out for himself—he is learning how to self-soothe. Once the baby does figure it out, he will be able to put himself to sleep without parental intervention. Remember, we all wake up through the night, turning around, pulling the blanket up, without noticing it.

While your baby is acquiring his sleep skills between 8–12 weeks, he has limited muscle response and does not have control over much. But it is imperative that you let your child find his own way.

If baby calms down at any point during the waiting period, start the clock again.

　✳ *EXAMPLE:* You are downstairs in the kitchen and hear the baby crying over the monitor. You look at the clock and see that it is 9:15 PM. If the baby stops crying at 9:17 PM, even for as little as 15 seconds, then you start the three-to-five-minute clock again at 9:17 PM.

✳ *EXAMPLE:* Wait another three to five minutes to give the baby a chance to calm down on his own until 9:22 PM. You should always use common sense.

If your baby calms down at 9:17 PM, but at 9:19 PM his crying escalates or you notice another negative change in the baby's cry (high-pitched screaming, wailing sobs, etc.), then go in and help the baby calm down before the three-to-five-minute time period has passed. Although your baby needs to find his own path to restful sleep, little is learned if the baby is completely out of control.

If baby is still crying after five minutes, go into the nursery, and reassure baby from the side of the crib without picking him up.

- Use your nighttime toolbox (see page 55).
- *Do not* talk to or make eye contact with your baby.

While it is a good thing to shush and whisper to your baby, do not speak to your baby in a conversational tone. Nighttime is sleep time and it is supposed to be boring and quiet. If you carry on a conversation with your baby, or look directly into his eyes while he lies in his crib, he might think he is missing out on something and may try to stay awake.

> ✳ *MULTIPLES:* If you are working with multiples, then you run the risk of a lively conversation waking up the other baby or babies.

Once baby settles down, step away from the crib, leave the room, and close the door behind you.

Once the baby is calm, he makes a quick inhaling noise or stops crying altogether. At this point, you want to step away from the crib and leave the room. From the moment he is calm, you want to leave him alone.

Wait another three to five minutes before going in again.

Remember, your role is to step in and take it down a level for the baby, but do not fix the problem for him by soothing him back to sleep.

You might have to repeat this process several times throughout the night. However, the frequency with which you have to go in to help your baby and the duration of each crying episode diminishes over time.

Many questions arise from Step 3, but the answers are usually the same: You are coaching your child to self-soothe at night so you should not do too much for him in this step. He is ready to soothe himself if you let him.

Here are some questions that I am frequently asked:

What if my baby does not sleep for twelve hours? What if she wakes up after only ten-and-a-half hours?

Each child will have a different sleep pattern. Some babies will sleep the entire twelve hours, while others might sleep ten to eleven hours and then be awake one to two hours. But your baby should stay in her crib either way. Your baby should wake up in a good mood and then entertain herself in her crib without crying until it is time to start the day. In other words, the baby should not wake and then immediately scream for the parents to run into the nursery to pick her up out of the crib.

You should treat crying during the last hours before the baby starts her day exactly as you would at any other point during the night: Give the baby three to five minutes to calm down on her own before going into the nursery to assist, and then leave the room once things settle down. Just because the baby is awake before the end of the twelve hours does not mean the baby gets to leave the crib. Otherwise, the baby, not the parent, is setting the schedule. Remember you are the parent; you are in charge. And quiet time in the crib actually teaches your baby wonderful skills, such as independent play and courteousness toward other family members.

Although my baby is sleeping, he seems restless, tossing and turning for several hours. What should I do?

If your baby is restless during sleep or wakes up frequently, try encouraging him in different directions until you find the right one. How do you know which direction to go in? I often tell the parents I work with, hey, whatever works for you, chances are, it will work for your baby.

Brainstorm by asking yourself, "How do I like to go to sleep?" Let's say you like to have a comforter. Now imagine yourself with no blanket, just a sheet on top of yourself. You might say, "Oh, no, I could not go to sleep like that. I need to have that. I need to have my comforter. I need to be warm." You know yourself. At some point down the line you identified a comforter as a requirement for sleep.

It is the exact same thing with babies. You need to look at what you and your spouse like, because more often than not, what you like is what the baby will like. Although the baby is going to grow into his own self, you are your past, and you are your family, genetically as well as environmentally.

So if you like to sleep on your right side, chances are, your baby will too. So try the right side; if he is cranky, try the other side. What about trying a different blanket? Some babies will sleep only on their stomachs, despite the "back to sleep" campaign. Some babies will pull the small SIDS-approved blankies right over their eyes before they fall asleep, no matter how many times their worried parents pull the blankies back down. Even if you adopted your baby, the general premise still holds true: Encourage your baby in different directions until you find the right one for him.

I have heard that swaddling is a great way to encourage your baby to sleep. What are your thoughts on swaddling my baby before I put her down for the night?

While some newborns love swaddling, many babies want more freedom to move around as they get older. I worked with one family who tried to get their baby to sleep in the crib with multiple towels and blankets around her so the baby would have the impression she was being held by a person. They did this with the best of intentions—they believed "If the baby feels something on her back, then she is going to think it is my arm or my hand and she is going to sleep." But the baby was already seven months old, so she had the ability to move around and find her own comfortable sleep position in the crib. The towels and blankets were acting like a straitjacket, preventing the baby from moving into a position in which she could sleep soundly. Once all the towels and blankets were removed from her crib, she turned toward her left side, her mom's favorite sleep position, and the baby was sleeping through the night within three days.

So while swaddling might work initially, I would not completely restrict a baby's movement in the crib, especially once they are about six weeks and older. Older babies have to figure out how they like to sleep on their own and they need freedom of movement to do this.

✳ STEP 4: ✳
Sleeping During the Day:
One-Hour Nap in the Morning and
Two-Hour Nap in the Afternoon

My approach to naps is similar to that for sleeping at night. Babies up to 18–24 months of age need to sleep every morning and afternoon. For some of their nap-time, they might chew on a soft book, look at a toy, or just have quiet time, but they need to stay in their cribs for the duration of their naps. Basically, babies need to slow down to catch up.

Daytime sleep training should begin about two

weeks after your baby is consistently sleeping through the night. At that point, you can observe your baby's natural sleep pattern during the day. You will then use this pattern to help set the naptimes. The baby should take about a one-hour nap in the morning and a two-hour nap in the afternoon, occurring at about the same times each day.

Like nighttime sleep, babies should nap in their cribs to further strengthen the association between the nursery and sleep. You should also use a "mini" version of your nighttime routine to signal to your baby that it is time to sleep.

Use some of the very same rituals you use at night: turn the lights off, draw the shades, play the same musical crib toy, etc. That way you will be sending a consistent message that these rituals equal sleep.

But do not feel compelled to repeat every part of your nighttime routine; a second bath or a clothing change is probably not necessary.

These naps should take place after your babies have eaten *and* after your babies have had playtime or another wake-time activity. The following sample daily schedule shows how eating, playing, and napping fit together:

Sample Daily Schedule

Time		Activity
6:45 AM–7:00 AM	😊	Wake, diaper change, dress baby
7:00 AM–7:30 AM	🍼	First feeding
7:30 AM–9:00 AM	😊	Activity Time
9:00 AM–10:00 AM	😴	Morning nap
10:00 AM–11:00 AM	😊	Floor time (tummy time)
11:00 AM–11:30 AM	🍼	Second feeding
11:30 AM–1:00 PM	😊	Activity time, outside if possible (walk in the park, stroller ride)
1:00 PM–3:00 PM	😴	Afternoon nap
3:00 PM–3:30 PM	🍼	Third feeding
3:30 PM–6:15 PM	😊	Activity time—very important to keep baby awake
6:15 PM–6:45 PM	😊	Nighttime routine before bedtime
6:45 PM–7:00 PM	🍼	Fourth feeding
7:00 PM–7:00 AM	😴	Baby goes to sleep in crib

The first nap should take place between the first and second feedings of the day, while the second nap should take place between the second and third feedings of the day. These naps generally take place two hours after the first feeding time and two hours after the second feeding time. However, you can modify this somewhat to fit your baby's natural sleep pattern and your family's schedule, so long as there is some wake-time between the feedings and the naps.

✳ *EXAMPLE:* If the first feeding time is at 7:00 AM, then the first nap would start at around 9:00 AM. If the second feeding time is at 11:00 AM, then the second nap would start at around 1:00 PM.

Your goal should be *no* naptime between the third and fourth feedings. Otherwise your babies will likely have trouble falling and staying asleep for twelve hours at night after the fourth feeding.

Try not to be too quiet during daytime sleep. While it is OK to draw the shades and close the door behind you to create a conducive sleeping environment inside the nursery, you do not want to create a noiseless environment outside the nursery. Everyday noise around the house actually is not bad, but good, during and after training. You want your babies to get used to sleeping through the phone ringing, the dog barking, and other normal daytime household noise. Remember, the babies need to adapt to the family's lifestyle, not the other way around.

Although you want to be fairly consistent in where and when your babies sleep, you also need to be somewhat flexible and listen to your babies. Your babies will have signals to tell you they are tired, so you can put them to sleep. Within reason, listen to these signals.

✳ *EXAMPLE:* The baby is not due for a nap until 10:00 AM but it is 9:45 AM and the baby is cranky and starting to close her eyes while she sucks on a pacifier. It is OK to put the baby down in her crib for her morning nap.

But if it is only 9:15 AM, I would try to soothe the baby with your daytime toolbox for 30 minutes or so and try to help the baby get closer to her target zone of 10:00 AM for the morning nap.

If your baby cries when you put her in her crib for a nap or wakes up crying during naptime, you should use the same methods you did to train your baby to sleep at night. For instance, if the baby wakes up halfway through her nap, give her three to five minutes to calm down on her own before going in to help her. If the baby is still crying after five minutes, go into the nursery and use the techniques from your toolbox to encourage her to go back to sleep on her own.

✳ *MULTIPLES*: It is important for multiples to go down for their naps together at the same times each day, just like they go to bed at the same time each night. And even though one baby may need less sleep than another baby, both babies should remain in their cribs for the entire naptime.

Chapter 5

Exceptions to the Rule

✳ How to Handle Changes in your Routine ✳

Once Baby Boot Camp (Weeks 8–12) is over, your baby will consistently sleep through the night and have scheduled feeding and naptimes during the day. While this is how your day will normally go, there will be days when there will be variations in your baby's schedule, both planned and unplanned.

Sickness

When your baby has a fever, a cold, an upset stomach, or another sickness, you should encourage your baby to stay within his schedule as much as possible. But you cannot expect the baby to follow his schedule completely if he is not getting enough rest or is in pain. Make the necessary adjustments and then return to the baby's regular routine once he is again capable. Reinforcement training may be necessary. Remember, it takes three days to create a bad habit, and seven days to break it. Be committed to breaking any bad habits that form while the baby is sick.

Special Events During the Day

For the first six months, I would try hard to stay within the schedule, even on the weekends. It is a trade-off, but a worthwhile one: The luxury of knowing that your days will be predictable and that you can count on several hours of free time comes at the price of working around your baby's naptimes and keeping your baby in a consistent routine.

Minimizing interruptions for the first six months

will allow the rhythm of the schedule to "set." A good analogy is Jell-O: Once the Jell-O has set for three to four hours, you can manipulate it by cutting it into cubes, layering it with whipped cream, or writing your name in it with a skewer. If you try to move the Jell-O before it has had time to gel, you will have a big, oozy mess on your hands. Likewise, if you try to introduce too much change into your baby's schedule before a solid routine is established, your baby will likely be a cranky, wriggly, tantrum-throwing mess too.

For the first six months, try to plan activities within their sleeping, eating, and wake times.

✳ *EXAMPLE:* Baby's four-month well visit with the pediatrician.

Your baby eats at 7:00 AM, 11:00 AM, 3:00 PM, and 7:00 PM. She naps from 9:00 AM to 10:00 AM in the morning and from around 1:00 PM to 3:00 PM in the afternoon. Eight AM is a good time to schedule the doctor's appointment and still keep your baby on track. Start feeding the baby between 6:45 AM and 7:00 AM, leave the house by 7:30 AM, and arrive at the doctor's office at 8:00 AM. Then the baby can have a half-hour appointment and still make it home for the 9:00 AM nap. If the doctor is running behind, the baby can, at worst, nap in the car on the way home.

Another possible doctor's appointment time is 4:30 PM. At 3:00 PM, you feed the baby at home, at 3:30 PM you change the diaper and get her into her car seat. Then leave the house by 4:00 PM. You have half an hour to travel and arrive for the baby's appointment at 4:30 PM. If you feed your baby away from home, i.e. in the waiting room of the doctor's office right before or right after your appointment, then you have even more options.

If schedule changes are necessary during the first six months, try to minimize the number of exceptions per week and try not to have too many exceptions in one day. Plan ahead and compensate when necessary.

✳ *EXAMPLE:* 2:00 PM birthday party.
Your baby usually takes his afternoon nap around 2:00 PM. Since that is the start of the birthday party, put the baby down for his

morning nap a half hour early and encourage him to take a longer nap then. Let the baby take a small nap in the car on the way to the birthday party, and don't wake him up for the first part of the birthday party if you can. Just let him sleep in his car seat.

Or you could let him sleep in the car on the way home from the party and even after you return home for a half hour or so. Then, comfort the baby with your daytime toolbox if he is cranky until bedtime. Remember, one day is the exception, not the rule. Your baby's rhythm might be thrown off that day, but as long as you stay within your schedule during the next two days the baby will stay on track overall.

After the first six months, going to a birthday party during naptime and other activities will have a lesser effect on your baby's ability to stay within his routine on the days following the activity.

Snow Days

If you lived in a temperate climate when you were younger, you probably have fond memories of snow days on which the weather was so bad that school was canceled or delayed one or two hours. Although a complete day off may be hard to come by, there may be mornings when you want to sleep past your normal 7:00 AM wake-up time on the weekend or even during the week. Or the baby is awake in her crib and you want to bring her into the "big" bed for a group snuggle. Or bedtime is at 8:00 PM, but you want to let the baby stay up until 9:00 PM to visit with her aunt and uncle from out of town.

After the baby has reached the six-month mark, it is OK to make these schedule alterations. But try to limit the alterations to one day.

✷ *EXAMPLE:* Sleeping in on Sunday morning
   You want to sleep in on Sunday mornings. The baby's first feeding is usually at 8:00 AM. On Sunday, try to sleep in until 9:00 AM and feed the baby one hour or so later than usual. I say "try," because your baby may decide a half hour extra is all he can do on some Sundays.

The baby is not going to forget his routine because you kept him in his crib an extra hour. But if you do it again on Monday and Tuesday, that is not OK—now it is becoming a habit that will have to be broken.

As your baby gets older, it is OK for him to "ask permission" for occasional schedule changes, like snuggling in his parents' bed, so long as he understands that it is a privilege, and if he breaks the rules surrounding the privilege, then the privilege will be taken away.

Vacations and Travel

Vacations and travel will produce the greatest disruptions to your daily routine. The first time is often challenging for the parent, because you worry that leaving the house overnight will create permanent havoc in your baby's life. Vacations do take children out of their routine, but it is important to stretch and find your boundaries as a parent.

Vacations are really just another example of the baby adjusting to the existing family unit. Although travel would be difficult during the Baby Boot Camp weeks, it is definitely feasible, especially after the first six months.

You will just need to prepare in advance and make the necessary adjustments. Bring a portable bed like a bassinet or a playpen. You will also need a room where you can do the nighttime routine and put your baby down for the night. But no matter how similar you make your home-away-from-home to your own home, your baby will not necessarily stay within her schedule. Think about yourself: For the first night or two, you may not sleep comfortably in your hotel bed or on your parents' inflatable bed, tossing and turning. But three or four days into it, you start to feel more comfortable because you have established a new rhythm away from home. Babies establish new routines while away from home as well.

Now, does this make your baby forget her home routine? No. She will adapt for a certain period of time, but after a while, she will start to miss her routine. We are creatures of habit. So if she gets cranky toward the end of your vacation, do not be surprised. Once she is back home, it may take a day or two to adjust back to her home routine, especially if you traveled to a different time zone. But she will snap back into it fairly quickly, so long as you reestablish the home routine with some reinforcement training, if necessary.

Mother Going Back to Work After Three Months

If you are using a daycare center, you might need to be more flexible with your daytime routine. Try to have the center incorporate your schedule if possible, but oftentimes they have their own routines established in order to care for multiple children simultaneously. If that is the case, follow the daycare center's routine for your baby on the weekends or days you care for your child yourself. However, keep the end-of-day and nighttime routines that you established during training the same.

If you have a nanny providing care in your home, then two weeks before you return to work, train your nanny to implement the same schedule you established. If you work together with your nanny during those two weeks, the transition to another caregiver will be easier for your baby as well.

What Should I Expect After Twelve Weeks?

One of the most important things to keep in mind is that parental reinforcement is a major key to long-term success. But even if there are relapses due to teething or other issues, it should not take more than three to seven days to get your baby back on track. In addition, this is the time to focus on naptimes and be as consistent as you can, especially until the baby is six months old.

Chapter 6

Extreme Circumstances

When I meet with a family for the first time, the parents often tell me that their baby has such unique problems that they fear the baby will never be able to sleep through the night. They feel that no one has it worse than they do.

I am here to tell you that there is no excuse for not training your baby to sleep through the night. Although each family and each baby vary, I have never met a baby I could not train using the methods described above. This list of extreme cases is meant to encourage you to tough it out—if they can do it, you can do it!

Extreme Colic

When I met April, her sons Adam and Aidan were sleeping super-propped-up in car seats every night with blankets tucked into every corner so they could not move. But the problem was that Adam and Aidan were not really sleeping in the car seats. They spent most of their time screaming.

Because they cried so badly, the parents thought that, when they did sleep, the car seats were the reason: "If I take the car seats away, they won't sleep anymore." I had to change the situation slowly because the babies had gotten used to sleeping in car seats. After several weeks of working with Adam and Aidan, both boys were sleeping in their cribs twelve hours a night on their stomachs with their bottoms in the air. That is how they liked to sleep. And the parents could not believe it.

Extreme Acid Reflux

I trained another set of twins, Brandon and Braden, who had extreme acid reflux that had been diagnosed by their doctors. They could not lie flat on their backs or stomachs for even two minutes without projectile vomiting and screaming. We still trained both boys to sleep twelve hours by twelve weeks in bouncy seats that were placed in their cribs. All other aspects of my plan, such as eating every four hours four times a day, no night feedings, napping twice a day, etc., were the same. By eight months of age, they were able to sleep twelve hours through the night flat on their backs in their cribs.

Cleft Palates

I trained a set of twins, Caitlyn and Carter, who were both born with cleft palates. This made sound sleep difficult because of the associated breathing problems. These twins were also sleeping through the night at twelve weeks. I did go back a couple of times after the twins had corrective surgeries at six months and ten months for reinforcement training, but within three days they were back on their twelve-hours-a-night track.

Quadruplets and Mental Retardation

About five years ago, I worked with a family who had quadruplets, two of whom had Down syndrome. All four babies were sleeping twelve hours through the night once they were over the nine-pound mark.

Constantly Held Baby

I worked with a set of triplets a while back, one girl and two boys. While the boys were sleeping through the night by 16 weeks, the girl, Diana, was not. She was the smallest of the three and had to be monitored closely when she first came home from the hospital. She also had a large birthmark on her face. Her parents felt sorry for her, and held her a lot. When the dad's mother arrived on the scene, she never put Diana down—she held her and held her and held her. While the other two babies were sleeping through the night, Diana would wake up crying after four to five hours. She could not calm herself and she would not go back to sleep unless she was held.

After the grandmother left, Diana's mother and I were able to train Diana to sleep through the night like her siblings, without being held, without crying continuously.

Human Pacifier

I had a client about two years ago whose eleven-month-old daughter Emma slept with her parents. Emma woke every two hours and cried until her mother let her breastfeed, or, should I say, snack on her boob. In essence, her mother had become a human pacifier in order to get some sleep herself.

Using the methods above, substituting a bottle for the breast between 7:00 PM and 7:00 AM, and having the father, not the mother, train the child for the first three days, Emma was sleeping through the night within one week.

Five-Year-Old Sleeping with His Mother

One of the most extreme cases I ever worked with was a little boy named Franklin. I interviewed with Franklin's family because his mom was expecting boy/girl twins. At the interview, his mom told me that, for two years, Franklin had been sleeping with her in the parents' bed while her husband, the dad, slept in the basement. When I asked why, she said, "Because that is what Franklin wants."

This went against everything I have tried to stress in this book: parental empowerment, the child adapting to the existing family, and the fact that children need, and thrive in, an environment with boundaries and limitations.

I told Franklin's mom that it would be very difficult and unfair to enforce two sets of rules: one for Franklin and one for his younger siblings.

So after the twins were sleeping twelve hours by twelve weeks, I moved on to tackle Franklin's sleeping issues. I was worried about success, because five is definitely the outer age limit on my skill in modifying bad sleep habits. But I am happy to report that after one gut-wrenching night filled with screaming, kicking, and a bedroom door with several holes in it, a new Franklin awoke seeking direction and guidance from his mother instead of dictating his own terms. Old rules had been broken and boundaries had been reestablished. Within a few more days, Franklin was sleeping in his own bed in his own room and dad had emerged from the basement.

Franklin's case did call for modification of my methods due to his age and the duration of his poor sleeping habits. But it should serve to inspire you to carry on with your own sleep training, even during the roughest of times.

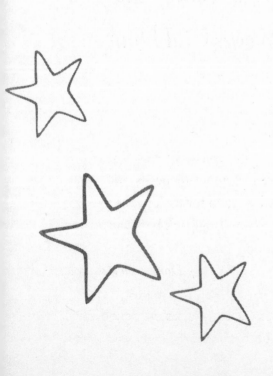

What Parents Say Who Have Used the Twelve Hours' Sleep by Twelve Weeks Old Plan

Suzy was the perfect baby coach for our family. She spent the time to get to know our needs and developed an approach that worked for us. Thanks to Suzy, I now look forward to my daughter's bedtime instead of dreading it.

— *Donna DePasquale*

We learned about Suzy shortly after we found out I was carrying twins. Our twins came early, and after a long hospital stay, they arrived home one week before their due date. Suzy helped us for several weeks after the twins came home.

When Suzy arrived at night, we always spent the first 30 minutes or so talking about how the day went and asking her for advice. What we learned in those 30 minutes helped us become the parents we are today. Suzy gave us practical lessons about raising our children that we employ each and every day. Our twins are now two years old.

First, Suzy helped us understand how important a schedule is for children. In fact, our kids thrive on their schedule—they know what to expect, and that gives them confidence and control. This is extra important in a household of multiples.

Second, Suzy put the decisions we were making about sleep in terms of how the decisions would best help our children in the long term. She taught us how to comfort our children and at the same time how to give them the tools to comfort themselves. Suzy taught us to think about the patterns we were setting up and how certain behaviors would impact our twins when they turned four and five. She taught us to value the things that would help our children grow with confidence and security.

Third, Suzy helped set up our bedtime rituals in a way that "valued" sleep. Our kids love their cribs, love to sleep, and welcome bedtime.

While there are still times when the kids don't want to go to bed, there are just as many times when they grab a hand and lead us up to their cribs.

Fourth, Suzy taught us that as parents, we are in charge. We set the rules, but we can create exceptions too. She taught us how to allow for flexibility without creating bad habits and what to do if we slipped and ended up with a problem.

— *Monica Dixon*

My husband and I have triplets. Suzy Giordano saved our sanity with her method of getting the babies to sleep through the night! Without Suzy's help, we wouldn't have lived to tell the tale!

— *Karen and Roger Mahach*

Being first-time parents at the age of 40, we had heard decades of children's bedtime horror stories from friends and family. With Suzy's method and loving routine, our preemie twins were sleeping through the night at the age of twelve weeks. Now, three years later, we STILL have perfect sleepers. They actually walk upstairs on their own, crawl into bed, and then call Daddy for their bedtime story. No getting out of bed, no crying, no need to make repeated visits to their room to reprimand or cajole them. No unhappiness at all. In fact, they have ALWAYS been very content to go to bed. They wake happy and well rested, ready to take on a new day!

The first night home from the hospital, we were so happy to have Suzy there to help us with our twins. Our original thought was that we could actually get "some" sleep at night, knowing that Suzy was tending to our babies' needs. We could not have imagined the impact on the long-term quality of our lives after Suzy taught our babies to sleep through the night by twelve weeks of age. There are no words to describe the gift she has given to our family. Now, three years later, her gift of struggle-free sleep remains with our happy, well-rested children.

—*Kelly Malesardi*

We had a shelf full of books about getting baby to sleep through the night, but none of them worked. The "cry it out" method seemed too cruel for us, and the gentler methods just didn't work. Then we heard about Suzy—and she produced a miracle. She taught our then nine-month-old daughter to sleep through the night in just three nights, with barely a whimper.

—*Dana Milbank*

Our now four-year-old twins have been great sleepers since they were infants, with the help of Suzy's sleeping strategies. From an early age, they were regularly sleeping ten to twelve hours a night and napping two to three hours a day, a fact that amazed our pediatrician.

Early on, it was a challenge to protect their sleep time, but we did it, knowing that it was the best thing for all of us. We always got them to bed on time, they were always home for their naps, and they were better behaved for it. Now that they are four, they have dropped naptime, but they still sleep about ten hours a night. They wake up happy, rested, and ready to start the day. Equally as important, my husband and I do too!

There have been only a handful of occasions when the children have slept with us, or vice versa, and that's when we have been away from home or when one of them has been really sick.

We are often complimented on how sweet and

well-behaved our kids are, and I really give a lot of credit for that to their good sleep habits. The early work with Suzy has paid off immensely for us. Not only did we get the sleep we so badly needed then, but we have two very well-adjusted kids who are rested, don't fight us at bedtime, and know when they're tired and they want to go to bed. There are so many challenges to parenting twins, but in our case, we are so thankful that sleeping hasn't been one of them!

— *Kathy Stokes Murray*

In addition to my twins, I am also the mother of a busy three-year-old boy. Because I had my other son to take care of, I could not nap when the twins napped, so I had to get my sleep at night. Because Suzy and her methods helped the babies sleep through the night so early, I was ready to care for all three of my kids each morning. I also exclusively breastfed my twins for eight months, and they were able to sleep through the night without any problems.

— *Molly Newberry*

I cannot begin to imagine how I could navigate mother-hood without the fundamentals I learned from Suzy

Giordano. She guided us through the madness of newborns. She trained our twins, born in 2001, to sleep twelve hours a night in just twelve weeks. She then trained our singleton, born in 2003, to sleep twelve hours a night in just nine-and-a-half weeks.

But even more importantly, we learned Suzy's extraordinary philosophy of raising peaceful, calm, confident, independent children. Our kids are no longer babies, and they have changed in thousands of ways since they spent their last nights with Suzy. But her advice has stood the test of time. They continue to thrive. Best of all, they know how to put themselves to sleep at night, calmly and happily. As Suzy says, this is a gift we have given them for the rest of their lives.

—Alexandra B. Stoddard

Upon learning I was pregnant with twins, the best advice my husband and I received was GET HELP AT NIGHT. My search led me to Suzy Giordano and hiring her was one of the best decisions we ever made.

Suzy was a big advocate of getting the twins on a schedule. She started working with us the first day we brought our new babies home from the hospital, and in less than three months, she had them both sleeping a solid twelve hours a night. She also helped us to become relaxed and confident new parents.

My husband and I joke that our family graduated from Suzy. There was much to learn on how to establish a schedule for the kids, but once we got it, it was great! We all worked together to put our newborn twins on a schedule that worked best for our family. What emerged was a sort of blueprint for the coming days and months of what we could expect as they grew. We were not at the mercy of a haphazard schedule. I felt that I could handle anything, and a confident mother is a happy one.

Having the kids on a schedule enabled me to go out with the babies by myself when they were just a few weeks old. We were soon in a playgroup, joined a gym, and would visit friends who also had young children. We were usually the only set of twins, and my kids were always the "good ones." Mothers with only one infant were amazed at how we were always on the go and wanted to know our secret.

My kids were rarely grumpy, always well-rested and, thanks to our schedule, I could easily anticipate their needs and adjust outings to fit around their feedings and naps. I could tell a friend to telephone me at three o'clock in the afternoon and be reasonably confident that both kids would be napping. This was very freeing.

There is nothing "easy" about having newborn twins, but having them on a schedule definitely gave us a good foundation. I cannot imagine what it would have been like with one child sleeping and the other needing to be fed—day in and day out. It certainly was an incentive to stick to the schedule! It was something that we had to teach ourselves as well as the babies, and for it to work, we had to stick with it. We did, and it was a positive experience that served us well throughout their early years. The children are now six, and have reaped the benefits of being on that schedule more than we'll ever know.

I look back at those first months with my new babies as happy and full of new and wonderful experiences—not sleep-deprived and stuck at home wondering when the next feeding would be. Most of this is due to Suzy's coaching. Her expertise on newborns is astounding. It was a learning experience that I consider a gift from her to both us and our kids.

—*Lisa Vogt*

Suzy Giordano is the mother of five children, the youngest being fraternal twin boys. Also known as the Baby Coach, Suzy has worked with Washington, D.C.–area families as a baby sleep specialist for the past ten years. She has trained hundreds of babies, from singletons to quadruplets, to sleep twelve hours a night. She resides in Northern Virginia with her family.

Lisa Abidin is the mother of girl/boy twins. She graduated with Highest Distinction from the University of Virginia's College of Arts and Sciences. After attending the University of Virginia's School of Law, she worked as a law clerk for the U.S. District Court and as a prosecutor for the Department of Justice. She resides in Northern Virginia with her family.

For more information, visit www.babycoach.net.

Acknowledgments

Many times throughout the years, I was approached to write a book about my methods and views on babies. But it always required me to take the time to do things that were just not "my thing," like keeping a journal. Then I met the Abidins.

As always, I had my evening chats with them when I first arrived at their home; we would talk about our lives, my philosophies, and, of course, babies. So when they suggested that I write a book, I said yes, and Michael took action. The very next evening, they said, "Let's start." Puzzled, I asked them,

"This is it? All I have to do is talk?" Michael smiled at me, and said, "Yep, let's talk." (I assure you, I do like to talk!)

So Michael, this book is here today in large part because of you. Thank you for starting us on it, for believing we could do it, for pushing us when we needed it, and for keeping us on track. And for supporting Lisa when she needed to step away from the "Mommy" role or the "wife" role so she could put all her energy into this project.

I share with you the success and gratitude of all who will use the advice in this book and feel better about the experience of parenting.

—Suzy Giordano